My Doctor Says I Have A Little DIABETES

MARTHA HOPE McCOOL, RN, CDE
SANDRA WOODRUFF, RD

D1114483

AVERY PUBLISHING GROUP

Garden City Park • New York

The information and advice presented in this book are based upon the training, research, and professional experiences of the authors. They are not intended as a substitute for professional medical advice. The publisher and authors urge you to consult your physician or other qualified health-care provider if you have any questions regarding a medical condition. Because there is always some risk involved, the authors and publisher cannot be responsible for any adverse effects or consequences resulting from the use of any of the suggestions or procedures described in this book.

Cover Design: Doug Brooks
Typesetter: Gary Rosenberg
Editor: Joan Taber Altieri
Printer: Paragon Press, Honesdale, PA

Avery Publishing Group
120 Old Broadway
Garden City Park, NY 11040
1–800–548–5757
www.averypublishing.com

The Diabetes Food Guide Pyramid on pages 46 to 47 was adapted from "The First Step in Diabetes Meal Planning" © 1997 by The American Diabetes Association and The American Dietetic Association. Reprinted with permission.

Library of Congress Cataloging-in-Publication Data
McCool, Martha Hope.
    My doctor says I have a little diabetes : a guide to understanding and controlling type 2, non-insulin-dependent diabetes / Martha Hope McCool, Sandra Woodruff.
        p. cm.
    Includes bibliographical references and index.
    ISBN 0-89529-860-0
    1. Non-insulin-dependent diabetes—Popular works. I. Woodruff, Sandra. II. Title.
    RC662.18.W66 1999
    616.4′62—dc21   98-51136
                                                CIP

Printed in the United States of America

10 9 8 7 6 5 4 3 2 1

Contents

Acknowledgments

This book combines information from both research and experience, and translates it into practical everyday advice for people living with diabetes. We would like to thank the American Association of Diabetes Educators, American Diabetes Association, American Dietetic Association, Association Diabète Québec, Canadian Diabetes Association, Canadian Dietetic Association, Juvenile Diabetes Foundation, National Institutes of Health, and Centers for Disease Control and Prevention for their ongoing efforts in diabetes research and the application of findings. These organizations make life better for millions of people with diabetes, and give hope for the future.

We would also like to acknowledge and thank Rudy Shur, Ken Rajman, Joanne Abrams, and Joan Altieri of Avery Publishing Group for their support and efforts in making this book a success. We sincerely appreciate all your work.

Our experience in working with people with diabetes has given us enormous insight into the problems faced by those who deal with this disease. We would like to recognize and honor our patients. Thank you for helping us understand what it is like to live with diabetes. You have made us better educators, enabling us to help many more people.

Finally, we would like to acknowledge our friends and family members for their enduring support and encouragement.

Introduction

The past several years have been eventful ones in diabetes research, producing many new treatment options for people with the disease. Improvements in technology combined with the development and approval of new diabetes medications have brought diabetes treatment to a level never before possible. Although there is still no cure, the treatments that are available today make it possible to exert more control over this condition than ever before.

Medical researchers have discovered that excellent diabetes care does indeed make a difference! The fact is that people who actively manage their diabetes and keep their blood glucose levels under control are far less likely to suffer from complications such as kidney damage, nerve damage, and blindness. But in order to manage diabetes, people with the disorder must understand what diabetes is and what the treatment regimens entail. What you don't know *can* hurt you.

This book was written to help people with type 2 diabetes learn the basics of diabetes and diabetes care so that they will be able to make wise decisions concerning their health care. Our focus is on the management of the most common form of diabetes, type 2 diabetes, which affects approximately 90 percent of people who have diabetes. In Chapter 1, we will review the underlying physical problems of diabetes and the different types of diabetes. In addition, we will discuss various approaches to treatment such as nutrition, exercise, blood glucose monitoring, and the use of diabetes medications.

Unless you check your blood glucose at home on a regular basis, there is no way you can be sure of how well you are controlling your diabetes from day to day. Chapter 2 explains the basics of home blood glucose monitoring and how you can use the results to improve diabetes control and prevent complications.

You may be surprised by some discoveries that have been made about the management of diabetes. For example, there's really no such thing as a "diabetic" diet. The truth is that people with diabetes should follow a balanced diet that includes a wide variety of foods—just as everyone should. Chapter 3 explores various approaches to meal planning and helps you find a diet you can live with. Regular exercise is equally as important as proper diet. In Chapter 4, you will discover the tremendous benefits of this simple and inexpensive diabetes therapy. You will be given general exercise recommendations and precautions. Most important, you will see that even a moderate amount of exercise can make a big difference in your diabetes management and overall health.

In Chapter 5, you will learn about diabetes pills and insulin and how they work to bring down blood glucose levels.

Is your blood glucose too high, or sometimes too low? Chapter 6 reviews the causes and symptoms of high and low blood glucose levels and explains the appropriate action to take in each situation. Most people with diabetes have been warned about the long-term complications brought about by ignoring their medical condition. This does not have to happen to you! Chapter 7 discusses the complications resulting from chronically high blood glucose levels. The emphasis, however, is on prevention.

Diabetes care presents unique challenges in special situations. The last chapter will discuss various ways of taking care of yourself on sick days and when you are traveling.

Although this book is loaded with information about the latest research on diabetes and diabetes care, it is not intended to take the place of regular checkups with a physician who is experienced in the care and treatment of people with diabetes. Everyone is unique. It is important that you and your physician work out a management plan that meets your specific needs. It is our hope that the information in this book will provide you with the knowledge you need in order to take excellent care of your diabetes.

CHAPTER ONE

What Is Diabetes?

"**Y**ou have diabetes." When you hear these words for the first time, terror begins to set in as questions race through your mind: "Will I have to take insulin shots?" "Will I go blind?" "Will my life ever be the same?" It's only natural to feel panic after learning that you have a condition such as diabetes, but your best defense is to calm down, take a deep breath, and be comforted with the knowledge that there are many things you can do to control your diabetes. Although diabetes will not go away, a few simple lifestyle changes can often greatly reduce its symptoms and decrease the risk of developing long-term complications. The first step in taking charge of your diabetes is to understand exactly what diabetes is and how it affects your body. In this chapter, you will learn about different kinds of diabetes and the risk factors for developing the disorder. Furthermore, you will realize that diabetes is a manageable condition. There are steps you can take to control its effects and lead a healthy, normal, and productive life.

DIABETES MELLITUS DEFINED

Diabetes, also known as *diabetes mellitus*, is a group of disorders that results in abnormally high *blood glucose*, or *blood sugar*, levels.

You will often hear these terms used interchangeably. Normally, when a person's blood glucose levels rise, the pancreas—a gland located just behind the stomach—secretes a hormone called *insulin,* which is used by the body to remove glucose from the bloodstream. The body uses glucose to produce energy. Any glucose that is not immediately used for energy is stored in the body's muscle cells and in the liver. But when someone has diabetes, either their pancreas does not make enough insulin or their body does not use insulin properly—or they have a combination of these two factors. This prevents glucose from entering the cells, which then become starved for energy. People who do not control their diabetes have elevated blood sugar levels, and this can lead to serious complications.

But what are blood sugar levels? To understand this, it will be helpful to know a little about the process of digestion. When we eat, a complex series of events is set in motion. As food moves from the mouth to the stomach to the intestines, it is systematically broken down, and carbohydrates, proteins, and fats are released. The breakdown of carbohydrates produces sugar. As blood sugar levels rise, the pancreas normally secretes extra insulin, which lowers blood sugar. If there is not enough insulin or if the insulin doesn't work properly, the glucose cannot enter the cells, and it remains in the bloodstream.

High levels of blood sugar can also occur if a person with diabetes has not eaten. Ordinarily, extra glucose produced by the liver is released into the bloodstream between meals as it is needed. Insulin usually controls this mechanism. But if the body has inadequate amounts of insulin, or if the insulin does not work as it should, the liver may release too much of this stored sugar into the bloodstream and cause blood sugar levels to rise.

Symptoms of Diabetes

Diabetes is called a *silent disease* because its symptoms are not always apparent. In fact, some estimate that only about half the people who suffer from the disease know that they have it. There are, however, some physical symptoms associated with chronically high blood sugar levels that can lead physicians to suspect the presence of diabetes. They can include some or all of the following:

- Excessive thirst and dry mouth

- Frequent urination with large volumes of urine

- Unexplained weight loss

- Increased appetite

- Exhaustion, lack of energy

- Blurred vision

- Recurring infections that are slow to heal

- Dry, itchy skin

- Nausea, vomiting, and abdominal pain

Symptoms of high blood sugar may appear gradually, or they may come on suddenly during any stage of life. In some cases, symptoms may not appear at all.

TYPES OF DIABETES

Although we speak of diabetes as a single illness, it must be pointed out that diabetes is a general term for a group of disorders that are related to the body's ability to process glucose. There are different types of diabetes, each of which is diagnosed according to the underlying physical causes of the problem. The three main types of diabetes are *type 1 diabetes*; *type 2 diabetes*—the focus of this book; and *gestational diabetes*.

Type 1 Diabetes

Type 1 diabetes, which used to be called *juvenile onset* diabetes or *insulin-dependent* diabetes, is a condition in which the pancreas produces either very small amounts of insulin or no insulin at all. According to medical statistics, less than 10 percent of people with diabetes have type 1 diabetes, and it usually strikes children and adolescents.

The onset of type 1 diabetes is usually swift and severe. Since people suffering from the disorder cannot make insulin, they cannot use glucose for fuel. Instead, their bodies must use stored fat for fuel. And as the stored fat is burned at increasing rates, toxic substances called *ketones* are produced. These acids build up in the body and can make a person extremely ill and can even cause death. The only recourse for people with type 1 diabetes is treatment with insulin injections. Without insulin, they will die.

After the diagnosis of type 1 diabetes, there may be a brief period, called the "honeymoon period," in which the body still produces some insulin. During this time—which is like a brief period of remission—reduced amounts of insulin or no insulin may be required. Unfortunately, this period is short-lived, and insulin injections must eventually be resumed in order to control blood glucose levels.

Type 2 Diabetes

Type 2 diabetes is by far the most common type of diabetes. It affects 90 percent of the 16 million Americans and 1.5 million Canadians who have diabetes. In the past, type 2 diabetes was called *non-insulin dependent* diabetes because people who have this condition still produce insulin and are often able to control their blood sugar without taking insulin injections.

The underlying cause is either decreased insulin production or, more commonly, cells that do not respond properly to insulin—a condition known as *insulin resistance*. Although the treatment of type 2 diabetes may call for diabetes pills or insulin injections in order to bring blood sugar levels under control, the preferred treatment involves a lifelong program of regular exercise, healthy diet, and weight control.

Gestational Diabetes

Gestational diabetes affects an estimated 3 to 4 percent of pregnant women. This type of diabetes is first recognized and diagnosed during pregnancy—usually, after the twenty-fourth week. If left untreated, gestational diabetes can cause the fetus to develop an overabundance of fat cells, resulting in high birth weight and associated problems during delivery. These infants have an increased chance of suffering from obesity later in life. Infants whose mothers have diabetes also have a higher risk of developing jaundice; and they may have temporary problems with low blood sugar and must be monitored and fed soon after birth. Uncontrolled high blood sugar in early pregnancy can cause birth defects.

During pregnancy, diabetic mothers may develop other health problems, such as high blood pressure, and they should be monitored closely by a health professional. Although gestational diabetes usually goes away after delivery, women who have this condition are at a higher risk of developing diabetes later in life.

Because blood glucose values in pregnant women are normally lower than they are in the rest of the population, the diagnostic criteria discussed later in this chapter do not apply to pregnant women. Therefore, all pregnant women who are at risk of developing gestational diabetes should be screened for glucose intolerance. A health-care professional can best determine who is at risk.

DIABETIC RISK FACTORS

The majority of people with type 2 diabetes develop the disease during adulthood, usually after the age of forty. How do you know if you are a candidate for the illness? There are definite risk factors, some of which can be avoided.

Diet and Lifestyle

Two of the strongest risk factors for developing type 2 diabetes are obesity and lack of exercise. It is estimated that over 80 percent of people who get type 2 diabetes are overweight. Many consume high-fat diets with a high concentration of refined foods, and they tend to have sedentary lifestyles. There is no question that positive changes in nutrition and exercise are often all that are needed to keep diabetes in check. The inset on page 10 will help you determine your ideal body weight. Chapter 3 provides more detailed information about diabetes and diet.

How does being overweight encourage the development of diabetes? As your body accumulates excess fat, your cells become increasingly resistant to the effects of insulin. Consequently, the pancreas must secrete more and more insulin in order to remove

Determining Your Ideal Body Weight

Excess weight is a powerful risk factor for developing diabetes. This is especially true if you carry your weight around your middle—if you have the so-called apple shape—instead of in your hips and thighs—if you're pear-shaped. By the same token, achieving and maintaining a healthy body weight is one of the single most effective strategies you can use to take control of your diabetes. In many cases, a sensible nutrition and exercise program that promotes gradual weight loss is all that is needed to keep diabetes in check.

How do you know what a healthy body weight is for you? One of the simplest means used by health professionals is the Body Mass Index (BMI), which describes body weight in relation to height. The following table will tell you your BMI at a glance.

Body Mass Index

BMI	20	21	22	23	24	25	26	27	28	29	30
Height					**Weight in Pounds**						
5'0"	102	107	112	117	122	127	132	138	143	148	153
5'1"	106	111	117	122	127	132	138	143	148	154	159
5'2"	109	114	120	125	130	135	141	146	152	158	163
5'3"	113	119	124	130	135	141	146	152	158	164	169
5'4"	117	123	129	135	141	146	152	158	164	170	176
5'5"	120	126	132	138	144	150	156	162	168	174	180
5'6"	124	131	137	143	149	156	162	168	174	180	187
5'7"	127	134	140	147	153	159	166	172	178	185	191
5'8"	132	139	145	152	158	165	172	178	185	191	198
5'9"	135	142	149	155	162	169	176	182	189	196	203
5'10"	140	147	154	161	168	175	182	189	196	203	210
5'11"	143	150	157	164	171	179	186	193	200	207	214
6'0"	148	155	162	170	177	185	192	199	207	214	221
6'1"	151	158	166	174	181	189	196	204	211	219	226
6'2"	156	164	171	179	187	195	203	210	218	226	234
6'3"	159	167	175	183	191	199	207	215	223	231	239
6'4"	164	172	181	189	197	205	214	222	230	238	246

If your height or weight is not listed in the Body Mass Index table, or if you want to know your exact BMI, you can use the following formula to determine your BMI. Simply multiply your weight in pounds by 705. Then divide the resulting figure by your height in inches squared. If you are using the metric system, simply divide your weight in kilograms by your height in meters squared.

So now you know your BMI. But what does it mean? In general, BMIs between 19 and 25 are associated with the longest, healthiest life spans. A BMI of 25 to 29.9 places you in the overweight category, and greatly raises your risk of developing health problems like diabetes, high blood pressure, and coronary heart disease. A BMI of 30 or more indicates an even more serious classification of obesity.

Realize that if you are very muscular and/or have dense bones, your BMI is like to be higher than the standards recommended. This does not mean that you are not healthy—quite the opposite, in fact. If you fall into this category, you can get a better idea of what your ideal body weight should be by having your percentage of body fat measured. A health professional such as an exercise physiologist or a nutritionist can do this for you. The body fat percentages associated with the lowest health risks are between 12 and 20 percent for men, and 20 to 30 percent for women, with the lower ends of these ranges being the most desirable.

Before making any final decision about your ideal body weight, consult your physician, dietitian, or diabetes educator. If you have been overweight for many years, a realistic body weight may be somewhat higher than the BMI norms presented above. But realize that if you can lose even a few pounds and maintain that loss, you will reap significant health benefits.

glucose from the bloodstream. As insulin resistance progresses, blood insulin levels become chronically elevated, and this condition can lead to diabetes.

In addition, insulin resistance raises the risk for cardiovascular disease. How? Chronically elevated insulin levels are associated with high blood pressure, decreased levels of heart-protective

HDL, or "good," cholesterol, and increased levels of LDL, or "bad," cholesterol and harmful fats known as *triglycerides*.

Can you do anything about insulin resistance? Yes. In most cases, simply losing weight is the best medicine. As body fat diminishes, insulin levels drop, greatly improving this condition. Exercise is equally vital because it makes cells more responsive to insulin, thus reducing the amount that the pancreas must churn out. Chapters 3 and 4 will help you implement the nutrition and exercise strategies that can help bring insulin resistance under control. Since losing only ten or twenty pounds can bring health benefits to many people, it's well worth the effort to get started!

Family and Gestational History

People with type 2 diabetes will sometimes have a family history of diabetes. African Americans, Hispanics, Native Americans, people of Aboriginal and First Nation descent in Canada, and some Asian and Pacific Islander groups are at greater risk of developing diabetes than other populations. In addition, women who have had gestational diabetes or who have given birth to a baby weighing more than 9 pounds, or 4.1 kilograms, are more likely to develop the disorder.

DIAGNOSING DIABETES

Because diabetes is not always accompanied by obvious symptoms, the only sure way to determine that a diabetic condition exists is to measure blood sugar levels. If these levels are too high, there is a strong probability that diabetes is the cause. However, the disorder must be diagnosed by a physician.

But what exactly is a normal blood sugar level? That depends partly on when the blood sugar level is measured—before or after eating. Doctors use three tests to determine if diabetes is present. The first, called the *fasting plasma glucose test* (FPG), is given after the patient has fasted for at least eight hours. The second is a *random plasma glucose test*, which may be done at any time without regard to the consumption of food or drink. The third, called the *oral glucose tolerance test* (OGTT), is administered after the patient

Test Results:
Milligrams Versus Millimoles

Most people have no idea of what their blood sugar, cholesterol, or triglyceride levels are. But once you have been diagnosed with diabetes, you will become keenly aware of these health indicators, as controlling their levels is an essential strategy for promoting optimal health and preventing long-term complications.

Americans are used to seeing their laboratory results for blood glucose, cholesterol, and triglycerides expressed in milligrams per deciliter (mg/dl), but the rest of the world uses a System of International Units (SI units). This system expresses laboratory results in millimoles per liter (mmol/L). In a move to be more consistent with the rest of the world, many American researchers and health professionals are now using SI units, and some American laboratories are beginning to provide their test results in these units, as well. If you would like to convert your own test results from one system to another, you can use the following conversion formulas, or you can turn to the conversion tables that begin on page 131.

Desired Conversion	Conversion Formula
To convert mg/dl glucose into mmol/L	Divide by 18
To convert mmol/L glucose into mg/dl	Multiply by 18
To convert mg/dl cholesterol into mmol/L	Divide by 38.7
To convert mmol/L cholesterol into mg/dl	Multiply by 38.7
To convert mg/dl triglycerides into mmol/L	Divide by 88.5

has ingested a special glucose-containing solution. Although each of these tests can be used to diagnose diabetes, the fasting plasma glucose test is the preferred method. Why? It is easy to administer, relatively convenient to take, and lower in cost than the OGTT.

If there is any doubt about hyperglycemia or the diagnosis of diabetes, a positive test for diagnosis of diabetes should be confirmed by repeat testing on a different day.

Fasting Plasma Glucose Test (FPG)

The fasting plasma glucose test is, as the name indicates, conducted after the patient has not ingested any calorie-containing food or drink for at least eight hours. A blood sample is taken in a laboratory or in the doctor's office, usually first thing in the morning.

In adults, blood sugar levels after fasting are normally less than 110 mg/dl. This means that there are 110 milligrams of glucose per deciliter of blood. Diabetes is diagnosed if the results of your FPG are 126 mg/dl—126 milligrams of sugar per deciliter of blood—or higher. Abnormal fasting blood sugar levels should be confirmed by repeat testing in a laboratory.

Fasting plasma glucose levels from 110 mg/dl to 126 mg/dl are considered abnormal and indicate a medical problem called *impaired fasting glucose*. This is a condition in which fasting glucose levels are abnormally high, but not quite high enough for diabetes to be diagnosed. Nonetheless, the condition should be monitored by periodic repeat testing.

Random Plasma Glucose Test

A random plasma glucose test may be administered at any time of the day, whether or not the person has had anything to eat or drink. This test is also called a *casual* plasma glucose test. Diabetes may be diagnosed if a person has symptoms of diabetes as well as random plasma glucose results of 200 mg/dl or higher. Abnormal test results should be confirmed through repeat testing on a different day.

Oral Glucose Tolerance Test (OGTT)

The presence of diabetes can also be determined by an oral glucose tolerance test (OGTT). The OGTT is not routinely used to diagnose diabetes. However, this test may be used if the results of the other tests are inconclusive or if the doctor suspects that gestational diabetes may be causing a rise in blood sugar. For this test, the patient drinks a fixed amount of glucose solution; then blood sugar levels are measured at set intervals.

Diabetes is diagnosed if results of an oral glucose tolerance test are 200 mg/dl or higher two hours after drinking the glucose solution. Test results of 140 mg/dl and over, but under 200 mg/dl, indicate that the body has a problem metabolizing glucose. This condition is called *impaired glucose tolerance*. Individuals with impaired glucose tolerance are not considered diabetic, but they are in danger of developing diabetes as well as cardiovascular disease. Studies show that a program of regular exercise, balanced meals, and weight management can delay or even prevent the onset of diabetes in these cases.

As you see, diagnostic tests for diabetes can be performed in various ways, and the results may reveal disorders other than diabetes. Equally important, testing can warn individuals that they are in danger of developing diabetes. In these cases, steps can be taken to stop the disease before it starts.

Recommendations for Type 2 Diabetes Testing

Testing for type 2 diabetes is extremely important, particularly if there are indications based on lifestyle or medical status that diabetes could be a threat. It is recommended that all people over the age of forty-five be tested for diabetes, even if they do not have symptoms of the disease. Testing should be repeated every three years. People with the following risk factors for diabetes should be tested at an earlier age and more often:

- Obesity—a BMI of 25 or more (see the inset on page 10).

- High-risk ethnic background, including: African American, Hispanic, Native American, Aboriginal and First Nation descent in Canada, and some Asian or Pacific Islander groups.

- An immediate family member with the disease.

- History of gestational diabetes or delivery of a baby weighing over 9 pounds.

- Hypertension—blood pressure greater than 140/90.

- HDL cholesterol level lower than or equal to 35 mg/dl.

- Triglyceride level higher than or equal to 250 mg/dl.

- History of either impaired glucose tolerance or impaired fasting glucose.

SOME COMMON MISCONCEPTIONS ABOUT DIABETES

Although there have been enormous advances and many changes in the treatment of diabetes in recent years, many inaccuracies about the disorder persist. In order to clarify matters, some common misconceptions are presented here, followed by information that will help dispel any misunderstanding you may have about diabetes.

- **"Diabetes that requires insulin is worse than diabetes that is controlled without insulin."**
  Although good nutrition and exercise are essential to diabetes management, you will need additional therapy if your blood sugar levels remain elevated. People with diabetes who keep their blood glucose under control—*whether or not they use insulin*—are much better off than those who allow their blood glucose levels to increase.

- **"Diabetes will go away."**
  You can control the symptoms of diabetes, but the underlying physical condition will not go away. It is important to keep in mind that you will have diabetes for the rest of your life, and you must take care of yourself properly in order to prevent complications.

- **"Once you take insulin, you will always have to take it."**
  People with type 1 diabetes must take insulin for the rest of their lives. People with type 2 diabetes may need insulin at different times in their lives—perhaps at the onset of diabetes to get blood sugar levels under control, during illness or periods of extreme stress, after surgery, or as the disease progresses later on in life. But they are often able to control their diabetes without insulin for a significant period of time—possibly for many years. Some people with diabetes may never need to take insulin.

- **"People with diabetes must have special foods."**
  Your diet should be well balanced and healthy, and it should include a wide variety of foods in reasonable portions. There is no need to purchase special foods if you have diabetes. Even favorite foods and recipes can be modified and incorporated into your meal plan.

- **"If you have diabetes, you can't have sugar."**
  People with diabetes must control sugar intake, but those who take measures to control their blood sugar can occasionally include sweets in their diet.

- **"There's a condition called borderline diabetes."**
  There is no such thing as borderline diabetes. Either you have diabetes or you don't. Problems such as impaired fasting glucose and impaired glucose tolerance, which we have discussed, can develop into diabetes. But they are not diabetic conditions per se, and they are often reversible with a program of weight control, proper nutrition, and regular exercise.

- **"Diabetes will make me lose my eyesight, get heart or kidney disease, etc."**
  Many people with diabetes are very healthy and do not suffer from complications related to their diabetes. Preventive health-care is important for everyone—especially those who have diabetic conditions. Taking positive action to adopt a healthy lifestyle will prevent many health-related problems. If problems do develop, it is important to catch them early.

MANAGING DIABETES

There is no doubt that type 2 diabetes can often be controlled by methods other than insulin injections. These include maintaining a balanced diet, getting regular exercise, and perhaps taking oral medication—topics that we will cover in later chapters. But there is yet another important element of diabetes management—coping with the denial, shock, fear, anger, guilt, and sadness that are common initial responses to the diagnosis of diabetes. You may experience feelings of loss—loss of control, loss of the ability to function, and loss of freedom. Your self-image and self-esteem may suffer. These emotions can overwhelm you and can prevent you from taking care of yourself. Fortunately, there is much you can do to cope with these feelings. You do not have to be at the mercy of diabetes.

Reduce Stress

It is common knowledge that stress has a negative effect on health. It is particularly dangerous for people with diabetes, because stress can diminish the body's ability to control the production and release of glucose into the bloodstream. For this reason, it is vital that people who have diabetes reduce stress in their lives. There are many ways this can be done. The following list offers some simple suggestions for reducing stress:

- Get plenty of rest and sleep.

- Eat regular, well-balanced meals.

- Exercise on a regular basis.

- Practice positive thinking.

- Take up a hobby or pastime that you enjoy.

- Learn to say "no" to anything that increases your stress level. Be aware that even things that you enjoy can be stressful if you are already too busy.

- Examine your lifestyle and consider ways to make things easier. Identify stressors that you can eliminate from your life. Get rid of clutter; organize your home and your life to reduce stress.

- Practice relaxation and deep breathing exercises.

- Seek counseling to help you identify other ways to combat stress.

- If finances are a worry, work with a financial advisor who can help you organize your bills. In addition, free seminars on topics such as Medicare and insurance coverage are often available.

As you begin to follow some of these suggestions, you will see immediate results in your sense of well-being and in your ability to control your diabetes. Make good emotional health a top priority.

Find Support

One of your first steps in learning to deal with diabetes should be to identify sources of practical and emotional assistance. Certainly, family and friends can provide invaluable emotional and psychological help from day to day, easing your adjustment to diabetes. But if your problems are sidetracking or worrying you excessively, there are other people who can help you deal with them. For emotional support, therapists or social workers can help you overcome feelings of anxiety or sadness, and they can help you open the door to a more positive, hopeful, and healthy life. There is help available, and you should take advantage of it.

A diabetes support group can also be helpful. In addition to providing an emotional brace, it will keep you informed about proper care and the latest findings in diabetes research. Talking to people who have a firsthand understanding of what you are going through may help you see things in a different light and assist you in creating new ways to deal with obstacles. Many communities have diabetes support groups. To find a group in your area, call the American Association of Diabetes Educators, the American Diabetes Association, or the Canadian Diabetes Association, and ask to be referred to a group in your community. You will find the telephone numbers of these organizations listed in the back of this book.

CONCLUSION

You are now armed with some basic information about diabetes and its management. More important, you are aware that there is a great deal that you can do to counteract and control the effects of this disease. You may not have to take insulin or medication for the rest of your life, and you can reduce your risk factors for major complications as a result of the disease. In the pages that follow, you will learn more about diabetes-related complications and how they can be avoided or alleviated.

CHAPTER TWO

Glucose Monitoring Made Easy

A lthough taking control of your diabetes is not always an easy task, it is well worth the effort. What you do today in terms of managing the disorder will affect your health and well-being for the rest of your life. One of the most important things you can do to keep your diabetes under control is to check your blood sugar level on a regular basis. In order to do this, you will need a blood glucose monitor, and you will need to know how to interpret your test results. This chapter will provide you with the information you need to get started.

WHAT SHOULD YOU LOOK FOR IN A MONITOR?

There is no need to make a special trip to a doctor or laboratory to get your blood sugar checked. Technological advances have made it easier than ever to check it at home. And there are now several excellent blood glucose monitoring systems available for home use, which may be purchased at a pharmacy with or without a prescription from your doctor.

Which of the available monitors would best meet your needs? Before buying a blood glucose monitor, check out the features available with different brands. You might also ask your doctor and diabetes educator which monitors they recommend and why they recommend them. And you might ask someone who uses a glucose monitor about their satisfaction with their particular brand. Finally, you can research consumer and trade magazines, which often test the reliability of monitors and other equipment.

Some specific considerations can help you decide which monitor to buy. The following checklist will serve as a useful guide.

- **What is the quality of the manufacturer's support for the consumer?** Most manufacturers of blood glucose monitors have a technical assistance line for consumer support. If you have problems with your monitor, you should be able to call the manufacturer's toll-free number for assistance twenty-four hours a day.

- **How much must you spend for the monitor and testing supplies?** Expensive monitors are not always the best. Look for a monitor that suits your individual needs.

- **What is the availability of supplies in your local pharmacy?**

- **Does your insurance company cover the brand you choose?** Some insurance companies will only reimburse for certain brands of monitors and supplies. Full or partial funding is available throughout most of Canada. You can get more information about reimbursement from the American Diabetes Association, the Canadian Diabetes Association, or your diabetes educator.

- **How complex is the test procedure?** Some monitors require fewer steps in the test procedure and are easier to use.

- **What are the maintenance requirements?** Some monitors require more maintenance than others do.

- **Do you have any physical problems that may make monitoring more difficult?** If you have problems with your hands, select a monitor with a simple test procedure. If you have vision problems, look for a monitor that displays large numbers that are easy to see. There are also monitors that give audible instructions throughout the test procedure.

- **Does the monitor have a memory function that stores test results?** This is a convenient feature if you sometimes forget your test results or are unable to write them down at the time you test. But even if your monitor has this feature, you should still write down your test results so that you can see patterns in your blood glucose control.

- **Does the monitoring system come with a quality-control test to help you determine if it is functioning correctly?** This usually includes a "check strip" and/or "control solution" with which you can test the accuracy of the monitoring system.

- **Does the monitoring system have an automatic timing feature?** Some monitors will automatically time the test as soon as you apply your blood to the test strip. This is a helpful feature because there is less room for error due to inaccurate timing. In general, it is desirable to stay away from monitoring systems that require you to time the test procedure and wipe the test strip. The more steps in the procedure, the more room there is for error.

Checking Your Monitor's Accuracy

You should check your monitoring system on a regular basis to make sure that it is working properly. Manufacturers' recommendations for frequency in checking will vary, but you should check it at least once a week and any time you suspect an error in test results. You should check your test strips every time you open a new package. Furthermore, whenever you make a change in your medication based on test results, you should check your system.

Monitors should come with all the necessary materials for testing the accuracy of the system. Most monitors have a control solution that is applied to one of the test strips. If the strips and monitor are reliable, the solution will produce test results within a certain range. If results fall outside the control range, there may have been an error in the test procedure or a problem with the test strips or monitor. Be sure to try a second time.

Don't use monitors or strips if they don't pass quality-control tests. Always follow the manufacturer's instructions for troubleshooting; or, if your need further assistance, call the toll-free number printed in the manual.

CHECKING YOUR BLOOD SUGAR LEVEL

You will have the greatest success in keeping your diabetes under control if you test your blood sugar at appropriate times; if you do all you can to get accurate results; and if you keep track of your results. The following sections will help you make blood glucose monitoring an effective part of your self-care program.

How Do You Check Blood Sugar?

No matter which monitor you select, there are standard procedures that you should follow when checking your blood glucose. Before getting started, always wash your hands with soap and warm water. This will help your blood vessels dilate, which will make it easier for you to get enough blood for the test. It is not necessary to clean your finger with alcohol. In fact, if the alcohol is not completely dry before you stick your finger, it may mix with the drop of blood you are sampling and influence the test results. So if you do use alcohol to clean your finger, be sure to let it dry completely.

Your monitor will come with a spring-loaded device and small needles, or *lancets*, which you will use to prick your finger. To obtain a drop of blood, put the device against the side of your fingertip and release the spring. It is important to use a different fingertip each time you test your blood sugar to avoid soreness and the buildup of calluses. Any finger may be used to obtain the sample of blood. If you prick the side of your fingertip, it is usually not as painful, and you will also get a larger drop of blood.

One of the most common errors in blood glucose testing is the failure to get a large enough drop of blood to sample. You should obtain a large hanging drop of blood that will cover the entire the test strip. Don't smear or dab the blood sample on the strip. If you have trouble getting enough blood, "milk" the finger from the hand down to the fingertip. Avoid squeezing the fingertip, because this can also cause errors in test results.

When Should You Check Blood Sugar?

How often you check your blood sugar depends on the type of diabetes you have, how motivated you are to control it, and how you control it—that is, through diet, exercise, or medication. Your blood glucose level will normally fluctuate according to your diet, activity level, medication, and other factors in your life. You must check your blood sugar more often during periods when you are neglectful of your diet and exercise routine, when changes are made in your diabetes therapy, and when you are experiencing significant changes in your health or lifestyle. The following section will give you some ideas about the best times to measure your blood sugar. Be sure to discuss this with your doctor or diabetes educator.

General Recommendations for Testing

Although you will be following a regular schedule for checking your blood glucose, there are times when it will be necessary to test blood glucose more often than usual. The following list offers general recommendations:

- If your blood sugar is out of control or if you are newly diagnosed with diabetes—whether you take diabetes pills, insulin, or control your condition through diet and exercise alone—check your blood sugar before each meal and before bedtime. Occasionally, check your blood sugar ninety minutes to two hours after meals and between 2:00 and 3:00 A.M. once or twice a week.

- Continue to test your blood sugar before meals and at bedtime until it is consistently within an acceptable range.

- If your blood sugar is consistently under good control, check it once or twice daily. In addition, check it at different times of the day on alternate days. For example, check before breakfast and supper one day, before lunch and bedtime another day, and occasionally after meals. At least once a week, check between 2:00 and 3:00 A.M.

- If you notice your blood sugar levels rising, or if you have problems with low blood sugar, increase the frequency of monitoring until you re-establish good control. During periods of illness and stress, you will have to check your blood sugar every three to four hours and follow specific guidelines. We will discuss this in detail in Chapter 8.

- If you take insulin, you should check your blood sugar twice a day at the very least, but preferably four times a day. Check it before each meal, at bedtime, and occasionally after meals to ensure adequate control at different times throughout the day.

- Checking your blood sugar before, during, and after exercise can be beneficial, and it can provide information to help you decide how to adjust your calories or medication for exercise. If you regularly measure your blood sugar after exercise, you will see the positive effects that exercise has on blood sugar control.

- Different foods will affect your blood glucose in different ways. You may find it useful to check your blood glucose after eating certain foods to determine how those foods have changed your blood glucose level.

Keeping Track of Your Blood Sugar

You will get the greatest benefit from your blood sugar testing if you keep records of your results in a self-care diary or a notebook. These results will help you identify patterns—for instance, frequent low morning blood glucose levels—and enable you and your doctor to adjust your care plan accordingly.

Your records will be most helpful to you if your entries include the date, and indicate the time of each test result in relation to meals. You may also want to note anything special or different that may have affected your blood sugar level. For instance, you may want to note that you exercised for twenty minutes in the morning. (See Figure 2.1 for sample logbook entries.) Because your daily activities can greatly affect your results, it is important to keep the whole picture in mind.

Finally, always remember that although a record of blood sugar test results can help you spot problems in your care plan, you should never change your medication plan on your own. *Always* consult your doctor before changing the timing or amounts of your medications.

Date	Breakfast Before/After	Lunch Before/After	Dinner Before/After	Bedtime	3:00 AM
10-1	75/162	136	148	101	
10-2	117	138	140/163	111	
10-3	109	133/165	141	115	95
10-4	102	119	152	120	

Figure 2.1. Glucose Monitoring Logbook

Goals for Blood Sugar Control

Generally, people with diabetes should try to maintain blood glucose levels as close to normal as possible. Nonetheless, some people with diabetes have more problems with low blood sugar, and it is appropriate for these people to keep their blood sugar levels a little higher than normal. You should determine your blood sugar goals with the help of your doctor and diabetes educator. Table 2.1, which was adapted from recommendations published by the American Diabetes Association and other sources, provides general guidelines for maintaining control of blood glucose.

Table 2.1. Goals for Blood Glucose Control

Time of Day	Normal	Goal	When to Take Action
Before Meals	Less than 115 mg/dl	80–120 mg/dl	If less than 80 mg/dl *or* over 140 mg/dl
Bedtime	Less than 120 mg/dl	100–140 mg/dl	If less than 100 mg/dl *or* over 160 mg/dl
1½ to 2 Hours After Meals	Less than 140 mg/dl	Less than 160 mg/dl	If more than 180 mg/dl

What Is HbA1c Testing?

There is another important blood test that you should have in addition to your regular blood glucose monitoring at home. It is the glycosylated hemoglobin test, or HbA1c test, which should be ordered by your doctor every three to six months. Glucose in the bloodstream attaches to the hemoglobin on red blood cells, and the amount of glucose attached to the cells can be measured. Your body replaces red blood cells about every ninety days, so your HbA1c test results reflect your average blood glucose for approximately three months preceding the test. This test is a better measure of overall control than a one-time blood glucose test.

Normal HbA1c test results are less than 6 percent — normal ranges may vary among laboratories. HbA1c results correlate with blood glucose values. For example, a score of 5 percent indicates an average blood glucose of 90 mg/dl (see chart below). In general, people with diabetes should strive to keep their HbA1c levels at about 7 percent or less. If HbA1c levels rise above 8 percent, additional measures should be taken to improve blood glucose control. The following table makes it easy to compare your HbA1c levels with your blood glucose levels.

Table 2.2. Comparison of HbA1c and Average Blood Glucose Levels

HbA1c	Level of Control	Blood Glucose (mg/dl)
5%	Excellent	90 mg/dl
6%	Excellent	120 mg/dl
7%	Good	150 mg/dl
8%	Acceptable	180 mg/dl
9%	Poor	210 mg/dl
10%	Poor	240 mg/dl
11%	Poor	270 mg/dl
12%	Poor	300 mg/dl

CONCLUSION

Home blood glucose monitoring is a tool that can help you manage your diabetes because it gives you feedback on a day-to-day basis. Most physicians and diabetes educators encourage patients to check their blood glucose at home. By doing this, you are acting as a partner in your diabetes management. In addition to keeping track of your blood glucose at home, tracking your HbA1$_c$ test results and other lab tests ordered by your doctor will help you determine improvement or deterioration in your overall level of blood glucose control and health. It is essential that you and your healthcare providers use the results of these tests to make appropriate adjustments in your diabetes care regimen.

CHAPTER THREE

A Diet You Can Live With

There is no doubt that a low-fat, balanced diet rich in vegetables, fruits, whole grains, and other wholesome foods is necessary for good health. It is absolutely vital for people who have diabetes. In fact, poor nutrition is a contributing factor for 90 percent of people who develop the disease. If this sounds impossible, consider that close to half the caloric intake of the average American is in the form of fats and refined sugars. And the rest of our diet often consists of refined grains and other nutrient-poor processed foods. Most Americans eat far too few fruits and vegetables and get only half the fiber needed for good health. When a poor diet is coupled with a sedentary lifestyle, the situation is ripe for the development of diabetes, obesity, cardiovascular disease, and cancer. Unfortunately, people in Canada and other industrialized countries are showing similar trends in diet and exercise habits, and this is contributing to an alarming rise in the incidence of diabetes worldwide.

The good news is that, in many cases, the right nutritional therapy combined with an exercise program is all you need to keep blood sugar levels in check. In this chapter, you will learn about the latest goals and guidelines for the nutritional treatment of type 2 diabetes. You will also discover how protein, carbohydrates, fats, and other nutrients affect diabetes. In addition to this important information, you will learn about meal-planning options that will make eating an enjoyable experience rather than a frustrating task. And finally, you will find plenty of helpful tips for handling special situations, such as eating away from home and dealing with sick days.

NEW THOUGHTS ON DIET AND DIABETES

Today's nutrition guidelines for treating diabetes are vastly different from those of even a few years ago. In the past, complicated, highly restrictive diets were the norm. In 1994, the American Diabetes Association revised its recommendations in recognition of the fact that no single diet approach is right for everyone. The new guidelines call for an individualized, flexible approach to meal planning.

Goals for Your Diet

Your diet should be planned with specific goals in mind. Naturally, you want to achieve a realistic and reasonable weight, but there are other equally important considerations. Specifically, your diet therapy should:

- Maintain blood glucose levels as close to normal as possible.

- Achieve healthy blood cholesterol and triglyceride levels.

- Prevent short-term complications such as hypoglycemia and hyperglycemia.

- Prevent long-term complications such as kidney disease, cardiovascular disease, and nerve damage.

- Improve overall health through optimal nutrition.

NUTRITION BASICS FOR TREATING TYPE 2 DIABETES

Good nutrition is the basis for the successful treatment of type 2 diabetes, and everyone with diabetes should meet with a registered dietitian or other qualified diabetes educator for help with the planning and implementation of a sound diet. First, it will be helpful for you to understand some of the principles upon which your diet will be based.

The Role of Protein

Protein, which is concentrated in meats, legumes, soy foods, eggs, and dairy products, is necessary for maintaining muscle mass, a healthy immune system, and many functions of the body. There are two reasons that people with diabetes should include a protein-rich food in every meal: first, protein helps keep you feeling full and satisfied—an important consideration for anyone following a weight-control program; and, second, a meal that contains protein as well as carbohydrates has a gentler effect on blood sugar than an exclusively carbohydrate-rich meal.

How much protein should you eat? It is believed that 10 to 20 percent of your calories should come from protein, an amount easily obtained by eating two to three servings of lean meat, legumes, or tofu and two to three servings of low-fat dairy products every day. People who have kidney disease—a common complication of diabetes—may have to restrict their protein to the lower end of this range. This is because a diet relatively low in protein saves wear and tear on the kidneys, which help dismantle and excrete excess protein from the body.

The Role of Carbohydrates

If protein makes up 10 to 20 percent of calories in the diet, that leaves 80 to 90 percent to be split between carbohydrates and fats. There is more than a little controversy about the percentage of carbohydrates a person with diabetes should eat. Over the past few years, one of the biggest changes concerning meal planning for diabetes had to do with the types and amount of carbohydrates recommended by health professionals.

A New Perspective on Sugar

In the past, it was widely believed that simple sugars—sucrose, or white table sugar—raised blood sugar levels more than the complex carbohydrates found in foods such as bread, rice, and potatoes. For this reason, people with diabetes were advised to choose starchy foods over sugars. However, over the past few decades, researchers studying the blood sugar-raising potential of various foods have disproved this notion. The fact is that foods such as milk and fruits, which are high in simple sugars, raise blood sugar levels less than most starches do. And sucrose raises blood sugar levels in a manner similar to that of bread, rice, and potatoes. (The Glycemic Index inset on page 35 presents more information on this subject.)

What does this mean in terms of your diet? It means that people with diabetes can include some sugar in their diets without adversely affecting their blood sugar levels. However, when including sugar or sugary foods such as honey, molasses, jellies, and desserts in your diet, it is vital that they are not eaten *in addition* to other carbohydrates. This is because foods eaten in excess of those prescribed by your meal plan can cause blood sugar levels to rise excessively.

In addition, you must keep in mind that although sugar allowances for diabetes are more liberal than they once were, sugar intake should be kept to a minimum. After all, it is still a nutrient-poor food. Eaten in excess, sugar can actually deplete your body of B vitamins, chromium, and other important nutrients needed to metabolize carbohydrates. And, of course, most sweets contain more than just sugar—fat and refined flour are usually the other main ingredients. These foods should not be a significant part of anyone's diet.

If it is okay to include some sugar in your diet, where do traditional "diabetic" sweeteners such as *fructose, sorbitol,* and *starch hydrolysates* fit in? These sweeteners, which are widely used in sugar-free "diabetic" desserts, produce smaller rises in blood glucose than do sugar, honey, and molasses. However, these sweeteners, which are chemically similar to sugar, do contain calories and carbohydrates that must be considered when planning your diet. It is the position of the American Diabetes Association and the Canadian Diabetes Association that these sweeteners offer no overall advantage to people with diabetes. In addition, large amounts of fructose may raise blood cholesterol levels; and

The Glycemic Index

The glycemic index is a method of ranking carbohydrate-containing foods according to their potential to raise blood sugar levels. It was developed as a general guide for carbohydrate-intolerant people to use in managing their condition. The index can be a useful tool for people with diabetes. Choosing foods that have a gentle effect on blood sugar can allow you to exert more control over your condition. And since these foods require the secretion of less insulin, they can also help reduce levels of harmful blood triglycerides and raise levels of beneficial HDL cholesterol.

Need another good reason to use the glycemic index? Low glycemic index foods tend to be filling and satisfying, so choosing them more often can help you meet your weight management goals. What causes some foods to have a low glycemic index and others to have a high index? Several factors are involved:

- *The molecular structure of the sugar or starch in food is one of the main factors affecting a food's glycemic index. For instance, fruits are high in fructose and milk is high in lactose, both of which have milder effects on blood sugar.*

- *The kind of fiber in a food also determines its glycemic index. Soluble fiber, which is abundant in oats, barley, legumes, and many fruits and vegetables, is particularly effective at slowing the digestion and absorption of food. This is one reason that oats, barley, and legumes have such a low glycemic index.*

- *The degree to which a food is processed can affect its glycemic index. When foods are processed, fiber is usually removed—for example, fresh apples made into juice, or whole grain wheat berries ground into flour. Processed foods such as these are more quickly digested and absorbed by the body. Thus, they can cause blood sugar levels to rise at a faster rate.*

How can carbohydrate-sensitive people use the glycemic index to their best advantage when planning meals and snacks? Start by choosing foods with low to moderate indexes—that is, foods that fall into a range between twenty-five and fifty—such as oats, barley, bulgur wheat, legumes, fruits, and low-fat dairy products. Be aware that individual responses to high carbohydrate foods can vary and that some people can be more liberal in their choices than others. Some experimentation will probably be necessary to find what works for you. By checking your blood sugar after meals, you can see how you respond to certain foods.

When you eat high glycemic index foods such as bread, rice, and potatoes, include them in moderate portions as part of a balanced meal. For instance, have a small baked potato at lunch or dinner, and combine it with a serving of lean meat or seafood, a fresh green salad or vegetable, some fruit, and a glass of low-fat milk. By combining a high glycemic index food with lower glycemic index foods in a meal, the index of the mixed meal will be lower than one containing a large serving of a high glycemic index food by itself.

The glycemic index is a valuable tool for controlling blood sugar. There is even evidence that a diet emphasizing high-fiber, low glycemic index foods can help prevent diabetes from ever developing in the first place. Researchers who tracked the eating habits of 65,000 women found that women who frequently consumed refined carbohydrates such as white bread, white rice, and sugar, were two and a half times more likely to develop diabetes than women who consumed fiber-rich diets with a low glycemic load.

Table 3.1 lists the glycemic index of some common foods when compared with pure glucose, whose glycemic index is 100:

Table 3.1. The Glycemic Index

Food	Glycemic Index	Food	Glycemic Index
Cereals:			
All Bran	42	Nutrigrain	66
Bran Buds	58	Oat bran	55
Bran Chex	58	Oatmeal (old fashioned)	49
Cheerios	74	Oatmeal (quick cooking)	65
Cornflakes	84	Puffed Wheat	74
Crispix	87	Rice Chex	89
Grapenuts	67	Shredded Wheat	69
Muesli	66	Total	76

Food	Glycemic Index	Food	Glycemic Index
Crackers:		White rice	72
Kavli Crispbread	65	Spaghetti (white)	55
Melba Toast	70	Spaghetti (wheat)	37
Rice cakes	82	French bread	95
Ryevita	69	Rye bread	65
Stoned Wheat Thins	67	Whole wheat bread	69
Dairy Products:		White bread	70
Skim milk	32	White bagel	72
Whole milk	27	Kaiser roll	73
Low-fat ice cream	50	**Legumes:**	
Sweetened low-fat yogurt	33	Baked beans	48
Unsweetened low-fat yogurt	14	Kidney beans	27
Fruits:		Black-eyed peas	42
Apples	36	Butterbeans	31
Apple juice	41	Chickpeas	33
Banana	53	Lentils	29
Cherries	22	Lima beans	32
Grapefruit	25	Navy beans	38
Grapefruit juice	48	Pinto beans	39
Oranges	43	Split peas	32
Orange juice	57	**Starchy Vegetables:**	
Peach	28	Corn	55
Pear	36	Baked potato	85
Pineapple	66	New potato	62
Plum	24	Parsnips	97
Raisins	64	Peas	48
Watermelon	72	Sweet potatoes	54
Grains and breads:		**Sugars:**	
Barley	25	Glucose	100
Buckwheat	54	Sucrose (white sugar)	65
Buglur wheat	48	Fructose	23
Millet	71	Lactose (milk sugar)	46
Brown rice	66	Honey	73

sorbitol and starch hydrolysates can have a laxative effect. Artificial sweeteners such as *aspartame, acesulfame K,* and *saccharin* are virtually calorie- and carbohydrate-free and are considered "free foods." Realize, though, that since the safety of artificial sweeteners remains controversial, it is best to use these products in moderation.

Benefits of Unrefined Carbohydrates

If you are interested in optimal health, you should make sure that unrefined carbohydrates—whole grains, vegetables, fruits, and legumes—make up the majority of your carbohydrate choices. These foods are rich in fiber, which promotes health in a number of ways. For instance, the soluble fibers found in oats, barley, legumes, and many fruits and vegetables help stabilize blood sugar levels by slowing down the rate at which food is digested and absorbed. Soluble fiber also fights cardiovascular disease—a common complication of diabetes—by reducing blood cholesterol.

Watching your weight? High-fiber foods are much more filling and satisfying than refined foods, so they promote weight loss. How much fiber should you eat? Aim for twenty to thirty-five grams per day—about twice the amount eaten by the average American.

Fiber isn't the only reason to eat whole grains, vegetables, fruits, and legumes, however. These foods offer a wide range of vitamins and minerals that can help improve blood glucose control. For instance, whole grains provide chromium, magnesium, zinc, and B vitamins, all of which help the body process carbohydrates. Many of these nutrients are lost when grains are refined.

Vegetables and fruits are also rich in *antioxidants*—substances that neutralize the destructive free radicals that damage cells and contribute to a myriad of health problems, including arthritis, cancer, and visual disorders such as cataracts and age-related degeneration of the retina. Antioxidants also help protect against cardiovascular disease, which is the major cause of death in people with diabetes. In addition, researchers are beginning to discover that these substances may help prevent damage to small blood vessels, which can cause complications such as blindness, kidney failure, and circulatory problems.

Need another reason to eat more vegetables, fruits, whole grains, and legumes? These foods are loaded with *phytochemicals*—health-promoting substances that occur naturally in a wide variety of plant foods. Scientists are just beginning to understand how these powerful chemicals work, but it is clear that many phyto-chemicals are potent antioxidants, and that they work in a variety of ways to help fight long-term diabetic complications, cancer, heart disease, and many other health problems.

How High Can Carbohydrate Intake Be?

The optimal carbohydrate intake for people with diabetes is still a matter of debate. Many researchers believe that people with dia-betes should follow the same dietary guidelines recommended for the general population—that is, a relatively high-carbohydrate, low-fat diet in which carbohydrates make up 55 to 60 percent of calories and fat makes up 20 to 30 percent of calories. The reason? This type of eating plan promotes weight loss and reduces the risk of developing cardiovascular disease.

The controversy centers on the fact that in some people, this type of diet has been found to increase the risk for cardiovascular disease by raising blood triglycerides and lowering HDL choles-terol. In addition, many people are not able to lower their blood sugar enough when eating such a high-carbohydrate diet.

So what is the solution? First, be sure that you are choosing mostly unrefined, high-fiber carbohydrate foods such as whole grains, legumes, vegetables, and fruits. You can use the glycemic index to help you select carbohydrate foods that have a milder effect on blood sugar. Second, be sure you are meeting your weight management goals. If you are overweight, cut calories enough to produce gradual weight loss. Remember that even losing ten or twenty pounds can bring about significant improvements in blood sugar and blood fats. These measures, along with a program of regular exercise, will allow most people with type 2 diabetes to fol-low the same low-fat dietary guidelines recommended for the gen-eral population.

As you see, there is no single solution that will meet everyone's needs. For some people with diabetes, a diet with a carbohydrate intake of 55 to 60 percent is perfect. For others, carbohydrate intake may have to be limited to about 45 percent of their diet. Your dieti-tian or other health-care provider will work with you to find the right amount of dietary carbohydrate and the right eating plan to suit your individual needs.

The Role of Fat

Although sugar and other carbohydrates get most of the attention in diabetes meal planning, excess fat is often equally problematic. High-fat diets are a primary cause of obesity, which is the underlying factor in most cases of type 2 diabetes. How do high-fat diets cause obesity? Fat is a concentrated source of calories that has more than twice the calories of carbohydrates and proteins. If you eat more calories than you burn, the excess will be stored as fat.

When planning the fat content of your diet, your dietitian will take into account your weight management goals along with your levels of blood sugar, cholesterol, and triglycerides. How much fat can you eat? In most cases, fat should make up less than 30 percent of your caloric intake.

In the interest of preventing cardiovascular disease, people with diabetes should avoid saturated fats—found in fatty meats, butter, hard margarine, and high-fat dairy products. Another type of fat to avoid is *trans fat*, a chemically altered fat that is formed when hydrogen is added to liquid vegetable oils to give them a more solid, buttery consistency. Like saturated fat, trans fat can raise blood cholesterol levels. You should avoid products which contain trans fat, such as margarine, solid shortening, hydrogenated vegetable oil, and foods made with these ingredients. Instead, emphasize heart-healthy monounsaturated fats, which are found in olive oil, canola oil, nuts, and avocados.

What About Alcohol?

Under most circumstances, moderate use of alcohol will not adversely affect the blood sugar levels of people who control their type 2 diabetes. How much alcohol can you have? No more than one drink per day for women or two drinks per day for men—one drink is defined as twelve ounces of beer, five ounces of wine, or one and a half ounces of 80 proof liquor.

If you take insulin, you should consume alcohol only with a

meal. Alcohol can intensify the blood sugar-lowering effects of insulin and cause hypoglycemia. Certain blood glucose-lowering medications can also react adversely with alcohol and make you very sick. So if you plan to include alcohol in your diet, even occasionally, be sure to check with your physician or diabetes educator for guidance.

If you are concerned about weight gain, remember that alcohol, like sugar, provides empty calories, and regular use of alcohol may slow or prevent weight loss. To keep calories under control, you can substitute an alcoholic beverage for two teaspoons of fat in your diet—the equivalent of 90 calories. To control calories even more, choose light beer, dry wine, or liquor mixed with seltzer rather than regular beer, sweet wine, and liquor mixed with a creamy or sweet mixer.

What About Sodium?

Type 2 diabetes raises the risk of developing high blood pressure, especially in people who are overweight. Some studies have shown that people with diabetes are more sensitive to the blood pressure-raising effects of sodium than people who do not have diabetes. How much salt can you have? It is prudent to limit your sodium intake to 2,400 milligrams per day. This is the equivalent of about one teaspoon of salt.

Remember that more than just sodium is involved in controlling blood pressure. For instance, diets rich in calcium, potassium, and magnesium can help reduce blood pressure. In fact, a recent study showed that people who adopt a low-fat diet rich in vegetables, fruits, and low-fat dairy products significantly lower their blood pressure in a matter of weeks. Many times, a healthy diet combined with exercise and moderate weight loss will eliminate the need for medications to lower blood pressure.

MEAL-PLANNING METHODS

These days, choice is the key word in meal planning for diabetes. Your approach to meal planning should be tailored to your individual needs based on your levels of blood sugar, cholesterol, and triglycerides as well as your body weight, lifestyle, and food preferences. The following section explores some common meal-planning approaches that are used to control type 2 diabetes. You and your health-care practitioner or registered dietitian will select the approach that best fits your needs. While these plans differ in their basic approaches, they all include the following guidelines:

- Choose healthy foods.

- Reduce caloric intake to promote *gradual* weight loss.

- Spread food intake throughout the day by eating three meals, with snacks in between if needed.

- Keep the carbohydrate content of meals and snacks as consistent as possible from day to day to minimize fluctuations in blood sugar.

- Incorporate regular exercise into your life.

Now, let's take a look at some of the meal-planning approaches that are available. Realize that it may take some experimentation to find the plan that best suits your needs.

Exchange Lists for Meal Planning

For decades, the most widely used approach to meal planning for people with diabetes has been the use of exchange lists. *Exchange Lists for Meal Planning* is a joint publication of the American Diabetes Association and the American Dietetic Association, which first appeared in 1950 and has been revised a few times over the years. The plan groups foods that are similar in nutritional content. These groups are called exchange lists because foods within each group can be exchanged, or substituted, for one another.

Most people with diabetes are familiar with the six exchange lists: Starches and Grains, Fruits, Milk, Vegetables, Meats and Meat Substitutes, and Fats. Each list presents foods along with their serving sizes, so that you can look them up and incorporate them into the meal plan prescribed by your dietitian. The ability to exchange foods within each list gives you flexibility in meal planning while keeping the amount of carbohydrates and other nutrients in your meals consistent from day to day.

By further categorizing foods containing like amounts of carbohydrate—for example, starch, fruit, and milk—and foods such as sweets and desserts into a larger Carbohydrate Group, exchange lists allow you to substitute foods from different lists without adversely affecting your blood sugar. For instance, if you wanted an extra slice of bread instead of a piece of fruit with your dinner, you could exchange one for the other, using the portions listed in each group as a guide. Or you could substitute a dessert for some of the starch, fruit, or milk in your meal plan. Just keep in mind that in the interest of nutritional balance, it is best to keep this practice to a minimum.

Aside from offering flexibility, *Exchange Lists for Meal Planning* helps you learn about the calorie, carbohydrate, protein, fat, and sodium content of foods while getting a balanced diet.

Healthy Food Choices

Healthy Food Choices is a joint publication of the American Diabetes Association and the American Dietetic Association. This convenient fold-out poster offers basic guidelines for healthy eating as well as simplified exchange lists. *Healthy Food Choices* can help you learn the foundations of healthy eating, weight management, carbohydrate counting, and meal planning. This plan is sometimes used as a first step to the more advanced exchange lists.

Carbohydrate Counting

An increasingly popular method of meal planning, carbohydrate counting is based on the rationale that carbohydrates are the main factor affecting blood sugar levels. How does carbohydrate counting work? It's very simple. You are allowed a certain number of carbohydrate grams per meal or snack. To make sure you stay within your carbohydrate budget, you keep track of how many carbohydrates you are eating by using a carbohydrate counter book, food labels, or exchange lists. As you become more sophisticated at carbohydrate counting, you will begin to understand more about the relationships among various foods, medications, and activities. And if you inject insulin, you will be able to make adjustments to your dose based on changes in your carbohydrate intake or activity.

Fat and Calorie Counting

One of the simplest ways to encourage weight loss is to count calories. This method can be a successful strategy for managing diabetes in some people. One advantage of counting fat and calories is that it encourages portion control, which is a great help for many people with type 2 diabetes—*remember that you can eat too much of the right things and gain weight.* Nevertheless, it must be remembered that just because your diet meets a particular fat and calorie goal, it is not necessarily well balanced or healthy.

USDA Food Guide Pyramid

A fundamental dietary guide for all Americans, the Food Guide Pyramid is based on six food groups: bread, rice, cereal, and pasta; vegetables; fruits; dairy products; meats and meat alternatives; fats, oils, and sweets. Grains, vegetables, and fruits are given the most space at the base of the pyramid, which indicates that they should be among the majority of your food choices. Meats and dairy products are next in line; and fats, oils, and sweets are given only a small space at the tip of the pyramid, which indicates that they should make up the smallest part of your diet.

Unfortunately, only one percent of Americans eat according to the specifications set forth by the Food Guide Pyramid. For most of us, fats, oils, and sweets make up nearly one-third of our food choices! As you can see, if your diet is "typical," bringing it in line with the Food Guide Pyramid recommendations can go a long way toward improving your health.

Canada's Food Guide to Healthy Eating

Canada's *Food Guide to Healthy Eating* is similar to the USDA food Guide Pyramid. Like the USDA's guide, grain products, vegetables, and fruits are emphasized; and foods such as fats and sweets are not featured at all, indicating that they should be used only in moderation. Most Canadians, like their American neighbors, could greatly improve their health just by implementing these simple guidelines.

Diabetes Food Guide Pyramid

Recognizing the simplicity and advantages offered by the USDA Food Guide Pyramid, the American Diabetes Association and the American Dietetic Association published *The First Step in Diabetes Meal Planning*. This tri-fold brochure opens up to form a large poster of the Diabetes Food Guide Pyramid, similar to the USDA Food Guide Pyramid. (See Figure 3.1.) However, instead of placing high carbohydrate foods such as potatoes, corn, and peas in the vegetable group, it places them in the same group as grains, beans, and breads. This makes it easier to plan meals that contain consistent amounts of carbohydrates. Your dietitian can adapt the Diabetes Food Guide Pyramid for you by prescribing the right number of servings from each food group to fit your calorie and carbohydrate needs.

High-Carbohydrate, High-Fiber (HCF) Diet

Developed in the 1970s by Dr. James Anderson at the University of Kentucky, this low-fat eating plan derives 10 to 15 percent of its calories from fat and aims for 30 grams of fiber per 1,000 calories. The HCF plan emphasizes unrefined foods such as whole grains, legumes, vegetables, and fruits. Lean meats and low-fat dairy products are included as well, but table fats and cooking fats are avoided.

The HFM Variation

The *high-fiber maintenance meal plan*, or *HFM*, is a more commonly used variation of this diet. It is similar to the HCF diet, but allows slightly more fat in the diet—20 to 25 percent of total calories. The fiber goal is 25 grams per 1,000 calories.

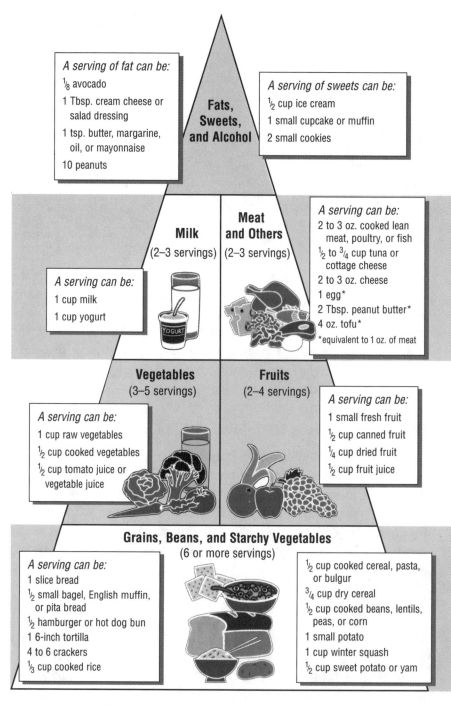

A serving of fat can be:

⅛ avocado

1 Tbsp. cream cheese or salad dressing

1 tsp. butter, margarine, oil, or mayonnaise

10 peanuts

Fats, Sweets, and Alcohol

A serving of sweets can be:

½ cup ice cream

1 small cupcake or muffin

2 small cookies

Milk
(2–3 servings)

Meat and Others
(2–3 servings)

A serving can be:

2 to 3 oz. cooked lean meat, poultry, or fish

½ to ¾ cup tuna or cottage cheese

2 to 3 oz. cheese

1 egg*

2 Tbsp. peanut butter*

4 oz. tofu*

*equivalent to 1 oz. of meat

A serving can be:

1 cup milk

1 cup yogurt

Vegetables
(3–5 servings)

Fruits
(2–4 servings)

A serving can be:

1 small fresh fruit

½ cup canned fruit

¼ cup dried fruit

½ cup fruit juice

A serving can be:

1 cup raw vegetables

½ cup cooked vegetables

½ cup tomato juice or vegetable juice

Grains, Beans, and Starchy Vegetables
(6 or more servings)

A serving can be:

1 slice bread

½ small bagel, English muffin, or pita bread

½ hamburger or hot dog bun

1 6-inch tortilla

4 to 6 crackers

⅓ cup cooked rice

½ cup cooked cereal, pasta, or bulgur

¾ cup dry cereal

½ cup cooked beans, lentils, peas, or corn

1 small potato

1 cup winter squash

½ cup sweet potato or yam

Figure 3.1. Diabetes Food Guide Pyramid

Diabetes Food Pyramid Guidelines

Fats:
- Eat less fat
- Eat less saturated fat. It is found in meat and animal products such as hamburger, cheese, bacon, and butter.
- Saturated fat is usually solid at room temperature.

Sweets:
- Choose sweets less often because they are high in fat and sugar.
- When you do eat sweets, make them part of your healthy diet. Don't eat them as extras.

Alcohol
- If you choose to drink alcohol, limit the amount and have it with a meal. Check with your health professional about a safe amount for you.

Milk:
- Choose low-fat or nonfat milk or yogurt.
- Yogurt has natural sugar in it. It can also have added sugar or artificial sweeteners. Yogurt with artificial sweeteners has fewer calories than yogurt with added sugar.

Meat and Others
- Choose fish and poultry more often. Remove the skin from chicken and turkey.
- Select lean cuts of beef, veal, pork, or wild game.
- Trim all visible fat from meat.
- Bake, roast, broil, grill, or boil instead of frying or adding fat.

Vegetables
- Choose fresh or frozen vegetables without added sauces, fats, or salt.
- Choose more dark green and deep yellow vegetables, such as spinach, broccoli, romaine, carrots, chilies, and peppers.

Fruits
- Choose whole fruits more often than juices. They have more fiber.
- Choose fruits and fruit juices without added sweeteners or syrups.
- Choose citrus fruits such as oranges, grapefruit, or tangerines.

Grains, Beans, and Starchy Vegetables
- Choose whole-grain foods such as whole-grain bread or crackers, tortillas, bran cereal, brown rice, or bulgur. They're nutritious and high in fiber.
- Choose beans as a good source of fiber.
- Use whole-wheat or other whole-grain flours in cooking and baking.
- Eat more low-fat breads such as bagels, tortillas, English muffins, and pita bread.
- For snacks, try pretzels or low-fat crackers.

How HCF and HFM Work

High-fiber, low-fat diets are very effective in lowering levels of blood glucose as well as cholesterol and triglycerides in many people. For some people, this diet can reduce or eliminate the need for insulin injections or diabetes pills. How do HCF diets work? First, fibrous whole foods such as whole grains, legumes, vegetables, and fruits are rich in magnesium, chromium, and zinc—nutrients that are processed out of refined foods. These nutrients help the body metabolize carbohydrates. Second, soluble fiber helps stabilize blood sugar levels. And, finally, high-fiber, low-fat diets promote weight loss.

The Advantages. A main advantage of the HCF and HFM diets is that they deliver an abundance of nutrients, antioxidants, and phytochemicals that can help prevent a wide range of health problems such as heart disease, cancer, hypertension, and premature aging. On the other hand, these are fairly structured diets, and some people find the dramatic change in food choices hard to follow. In addition, many people suffer from bloating and gas when adding large amounts of fiber to their diets. Nonetheless, these side effects can be minimized by increasing your fiber intake gradually and by drinking plenty of water. Once you become accustomed to a higher fiber intake, the side effects generally go away.

Month of Meals

Month of Meals is a series of menu-planning books developed by the American Diabetes Association. Each book offers twenty-eight days of complete, balanced menus for breakfast, lunch, dinner, and snacks. Recipes for many of the menu items and helpful eating tips are also included. The menus can be adjusted to meet a variety of calorie needs. And since each breakfast, lunch, and dinner provides about the same number of calories and carbohydrates, people can mix and match meals to suit their tastes.

People who desire pre-printed menus that take the guesswork out of meal planning often use this approach. It is a simple and flexible approach that does not require knowledge of more complicated concepts.

Individualized Menus

In this meal-planning method, your registered dietitian will work with you to prepare menus that specify which foods you should choose and how much you should eat at each meal. Like the other meal-planning approaches in this chapter, individualized menus are based on your weight-management goals, blood sugar levels, and blood cholesterol and triglyceride levels. And because the menus are individualized, they focus as much as possible on your food preferences and lifestyle. The menus may be very specific or they may involve some choices. No rules govern this approach to meal planning. You are not expected to follow the menus forever. Rather, you should use them as a tool to learn how to select foods and control portion sizes.

SUPERMARKET STRATEGIES FOR CONTROLLING DIABETES

As you work with your dietitian and physician, you will discover the eating plan that best fits your lifestyle and personal health goals. But no matter which dietary approach you adopt, you must still choose wholesome and healthy foods and avoid harmful fats.

Which Meats Should You Choose?

There are many low-fat cuts of meat from which to choose. From the red meat category, you can opt for top round, eye round, or sirloin. Otherwise you can select lean cuts of pork, such as tenderloin or loin chops, skinless poultry, and all kinds of fish and seafood. This will help you control calories and avoid artery-clogging saturated fats. Be sure to bake, grill, roast, stew, stir-fry, and oven-fry meats, seafood, and poultry instead of frying them in fat.

If you like ground beef and turkey products, be sure that they are at least 93 to 95 percent lean. If the package is not labeled, select ground beef that is the darkest in color, as this will be the leanest. Be aware that color does not always indicate the leanness of ground turkey, because various proportions of white meat, dark meat, skin, and fat may be included in the mixture.

Select lean lunch meats, bacon, ham, and other processed meats. Many products are now available that are 95 to 98 percent lean, and some brands are even fat-free. These products will save you lots of fat and calories. But remember that they are still high in sodium, so use them in moderation.

Meat Alternatives

If you prefer to avoid or cut down on your consumption of meat, you can experiment with ground meat alternatives such as recipe crumbles, tofu, or texturized vegetable protein. These healthy products can easily replace half the ground meat in chili, tacos, sloppy joes, and other recipes with little detectable difference. You can find these products in your supermarket or health food store.

Legumes are an excellent substitute for meats. Compared to other carbohydrate-rich foods, legumes raise blood sugar very little. (Refer to the Glycemic Index on page 36.) They are also exceptionally high in fiber and nutrients, practically fat-free, and contain no cholesterol.

Eggs and Dairy Products

Eggs are loaded with cholesterol. Just one large egg uses up two-thirds of your daily cholesterol budget. It also contains five grams of fat. This may not seem like all that much until you consider that a three-egg omelet contains fifteen grams of fat—and that's without counting the cheese filling or the butter used in the skillet. Fortunately, you need not eliminate eggs from your diet. Simply switch to a fat- and cholesterol-free egg substitute. These products allow you to create light versions of all your favorite egg dishes, including omelets, French toast, quiches, casseroles, and custards. Or try using more egg whites and less yolks.

As for diary products, there are now plenty of delicious ways to get your calcium with far less fat and calories. Choose skim or 1 percent low-fat milk, nonfat and reduced-fat cheeses, and nonfat or light sour cream and yogurt.

Breads and Cereals

The best grain products are whole grains. You can find a large variety of great tasting whole-grain breads and cereals at the super-market and at the health food store. Look for 100 percent whole wheat bread, whole wheat and bran cereals, oatmeal and oat bran, brown rice, wild rice, barley, bulgur wheat, and buckwheat. These foods provide fiber, antioxidants, phytochemicals, and nutrients that help control blood sugar and prevent long-term complications. Virtually all these health-protective substances are lost when grains are refined.

Fruits and Vegetables

Fresh fruits and vegetables are absolutely essential to your good health. Stock up on plenty of fresh vegetables and fruits. These foods provide fiber, antioxidants, phytochemicals, and nutrients that help control blood sugar and prevent long-term complications.

Fats

Some intake of fat is necessary for a well-balanced diet. But you must select the right kinds of fats and you must use them in moderation. When you use cooking oils, try olive or canola oil. These oils are rich in heart-healthy monounsaturated fats and low in saturated fats. When you wish to avoid fats, use non-stick cooking sprays for cooking and baking.

In addition, be sure to select reduced-fat and nonfat margarine, salad dressing, and mayonnaise. When you use these products in recipes and at the table, you can trim an astounding amount of fat and calories from your diet.

Snacks

When you're in the mood for a snack, choose low-fat snack foods such as popcorn, baked potato chips, baked tortilla chips, and whole wheat pretzels. For cookies, choose those that are lower in sugar and fat such as graham crackers and vanilla wafers. Low-fat ice cream, angel food cake, and low-fat pound cake are examples of other treats that can be enjoyed in moderation.

Always keep in mind that "diabetic" cookies, candies, ice cream, and other desserts may not be any better than traditional versions. When shopping for food, compare products for calories, total carbohydrate, and fat, and make your buying decision accordingly.

Looking at Labels

Food package labels provide a wealth of important information that can help you make wise food choices. First, check the label for calorie and fat content. Then, look at the serving size to see if it is what you would call a serving. (It's possible that your portion size is more than double the label's serving size!) This will allow you to evaluate how well the food follows the guidelines for fat and calories established by your dietitian and physician.

It is just as important to read labels for carbohydrate content. Many people look only at the grams of sugar per serving, but the total amount of carbohydrates per serving is the more important factor in how a food will affect your blood sugar. For instance, a serving of fat-free cookies may contain only ten grams of sugar, but twenty-four grams of total carbohydrate.

Finally, check the label for sodium content, keeping in mind that you should aim for no more than 2,400 milligrams per day. And look at the fiber content, keeping in mind that a healthy goal is 25 to 35 milligrams daily.

HAVING IT YOUR WAY IN RESTAURANTS

Many people find that they can easily master diabetes-menu planning at home, where they have more control over their food choices. But take these people out of their healthy home environment, and things can change dramatically. The fact is that the challenge of eating out can leave many people feeling confused and helpless. What can you do? Plenty. A growing number of establishments are keeping up with consumer demand for healthy foods. But even if a restaurant doesn't have any special low-fat or healthy items, there are many strategies you can use to make sure you get what you want when you dine out. The following tips can help make dining out a relaxing and enjoyable experience rather than a diet-busting exercise in frustration.

❑ **Plan Ahead**

• If you take insulin or a blood glucose-lowering medication, be sure to make plans for taking your medication on time.

• If you will be eating later than usual, have a small snack in the late afternoon before you go out to eat. This will prevent hypoglycemia and take the edge off your hunger, so you'll have more control when ordering.

• Call ahead to ask about the menu, or review the menu posted on the outside window. Also check to see if the restaurant honors special requests, such as broiling without butter.

❑ **Make the Most of the Menu**

• Request that sauces, dressings, and margarine or butter be served on the side so that you can control the amount used.

• Look for menu items that are steamed, broiled, blackened, grilled, roasted, en papillote, stir-fried, stewed, braised, or in their own juices.

• Avoid menu items served in butter, cream, or cheese sauce; marinated in oil; or fried. Beware of foods that are described as flaky, crispy, creamy, au gratin, battered, or breaded—these terms usually indicate the use of high-fat ingredients in cooking.

• Be creative when ordering. Consider ordering an à la carte meal—perhaps an appetizer, soup, and salad, rather than a full-course meal.

• If portions are large, consider splitting an entrée; or take half the meal home.

• When ordering breakfast, be aware that many restaurants now offer fat-free egg substitutes for scrambled eggs and omelets. Canadian bacon is a lean option for a breakfast meat.

• When ordering sandwiches, avoid those made with tuna, chicken, or egg salad, which are usually loaded with full-fat mayonnaise. Instead of ordering fatty cold cuts, opt for turkey breast, grilled chicken, grilled fish, lean ham, or roast beef on whole grain bread piled high with plenty of veggies. Hold the mayo and ask for mustard or low-fat ranch dressing as a spread.

- At fast food restaurants, avoid super-size, jumbo, and deluxe items, which tend to be loaded with fat and calories. Instead, order a small burger, roast beef sandwich, or grilled chicken sandwich. Grilled chicken salads, chicken soft tacos, bean burritos, and chili are other smart choices. Ask for special sauces, mayonnaise, dressings, and other toppings on the side.

❑ Other Tips and Tricks

- If you sit at the bar while waiting for your table, order mineral water, diet soda, seltzer water, or tomato juice.

- If you plan on having alcohol, use the guidelines on page 40. And remember, don't drink alcohol on an empty stomach!

- If you are prone to overindulgence, be the first to order so that foods chosen by others won't entice you.

- If you are tempted by the basket of bread that your server brings to the table before dinner, push it to the other side of the table, or ask your server to remove it. Nibbling on bread while waiting for your meal can cause you to blow your carbohydrate budget before the meal even arrives!

- When you are comfortably full, stop eating. Put your napkin on the table to signal the server to remove your plate This will prevent you from nibbling the remaining food on your plate.

Dining out is an important part of many people's lives. There is no reason to avoid it just because you have diabetes. As you have seen, with a little thought, it is possible to enjoy the pleasures of dining out and still maintain good diabetes control.

BALANCING MEALS AND MEDICATIONS

If you take insulin injections or a blood sugar-lowering medication, it is especially important that you take your medications as directed and then eat within the proper time frame. The reason? If you take an insulin injection or a blood glucose-lowering medication and you don't eat soon enough afterwards—or if you don't eat enough food—you can develop severe hypoglycemia.

If you know that a meal is going to be delayed for at least one hour, and changing the time of your medication or insulin injection is not an option, you should eat about fifteen grams of carbohydrate (for instance, one piece of bread, one-half cup of juice, or a glass of skim milk) at your usual meal time. This should be sufficient to prevent hypoglycemia. If you go too long without food and develop hypoglycemia, you must treat it immediately by eating a carbohydrate-containing food. Chapter 6 presents complete guidelines for treating hypoglycemia.

EATING WHEN YOU'RE NOT FEELING WELL

When you are sick, the last thing you want to think about is your diet. In fact, you may not want to eat at all. If you have diabetes, being sick with a cold or the flu presents special challenges—especially if you take diabetes pills or insulin—and you must learn how to cope with them. Chapter 8 offers suggestions about dealing with sick days in general. The following guidelines will help you manage your diet when you're sick.

- Eat your usual amount of carbohydrate, divided into smaller meals and snacks if necessary.

- If you cannot tolerate solid foods, you must substitute liquids such as fruit juice or gelatin dessert, or semi-solid foods such as applesauce or pudding. Try to keep the carbohydrate content of your diet as close to that of your regular diet as possible.

- Drink plenty of fluids to prevent dehydration.

- Know when to call your doctor.

The following table will help you select nourishment on those days when you are not feeling well:

Table 3.2. Suggested Beverages and Foods for Sick Days

Beverages	Amount	Carbohydrate (grams)
Apple juice (unsweetened)	1 cup	30
Broth	1 cup	1
Cola (regular)	1 cup	28
Cranberry juice cocktail	1 cup	36
Gatorade	1 cup	15
Ginger Ale (regular)	1 cup	21
Grape juice (unsweetened)	1 cup	38
Grapefruit juice (unsweetened)	1 cup	22
Orange juice (unsweetened)	1 cup	26
Pineapple juice (unsweetened)	1 cup	34
Skim milk	1 cup	12
Tomato juice	1 cup	10

Foods	Amount	Carbohydrate (grams)
Applesauce (unsweetened)	1 cup	28
Chicken noodle soup	1 cup	9
Cream soup	1 cup	15
Frozen yogurt or low-fat ice cream	½ cup	18
Gelatin (regular)	1 cup	32
Honey	1 tbs.	16
Oatmeal	1 cup	25
Pudding (regular)	½ cup	30
Pudding (sugar-free)	½ cup	16
Saltines	6 crackers	15
Sherbet	½ cup	30
Tomato soup (with water)	1 cup	16
Vegetable soup	1 cup	12

CONCLUSION

Diet is one of the most powerful tools you have to take charge of your diabetes. In fact, many people could greatly reduce or even eliminate the need for oral diabetes medication or insulin injections simply by adopting a healthy diet and a regular exercise program. Smart food choices can also help prevent long-term complications and greatly improve the quality of your everyday life.

There are many meal-planning options for people with diabetes. The kinds of foods you will be eating are the same foods recommended to anyone who wants to live a healthy life. Special diet foods are *not* required. This makes it easier than ever to find an eating plan that will fit your lifestyle, help you maintain a healthy body weight, and keep blood sugar, triglyceride, and cholesterol levels under control.

CHAPTER FOUR

Enhancing Your Life With Exercise

Someone once said that diet is a four-letter word, and exercise is an eight-letter word, so it's twice as bad. Unfortunately, this sentiment is all too common. Exercise can be an extremely enjoyable and rewarding activity if it is done properly and if it is slowly and consistently incorporated into your life. And there is no question that its benefits can be lifesaving. This chapter will discuss some of the advantages of following a program of regular exercise, help you choose a program suited to your needs, and give you advice about how to get started.

WHY EXERCISE?

Exercise is beneficial to everyone. It enhances the quality of people's lives by increasing energy levels, building endurance and strength, and increasing cardiovascular output. In addition, it releases natural chemicals called *endorphins* into the blood, which make people feel good and can give them a more positive attitude about life. People who have diabetes can reap even greater benefits by exercising regularly.

- Exercise improves blood sugar control. Your body burns sugar for fuel. When you exercise, your body uses more fuel, which reduces the amount of sugar in your bloodstream. Exercise also improves blood sugar control by helping your body use insulin more efficiently.

- Exercise improves weight control and results in better body composition. Because you burn extra calories and fat when you exercise, your body loses fat and increases in muscle mass.

- Exercise improves cardiovascular functioning. Regular exercise can lower cholesterol and triglyceride levels. It can also help control high blood pressure and decrease clotting in the blood. With regular exercise, the heart muscle becomes stronger, which reduces the risk for cardiovascular diseases.

- Exercise can be a good outlet for stress. In addition, it has an energizing effect; and when you feel good, your mental outlook usually improves.

There are many types of exercises from which to choose; you are not restricted to only one type of exercise. In fact, your exercise program is more likely to be successful if it includes a wide variety of enjoyable activities.

WHAT SORTS OF EXERCISES ARE THERE?

Exercises may be grouped into two broad categories, *aerobic* and *anaerobic*, or non-aerobic. Aerobic means "with oxygen." Aerobic exercises are vigorous exercises that require the body to use increased amounts of oxygen, which makes the heart and lungs work harder. This, in turn, strengthens the heart and lungs and improves their functioning. Anaerobic means "without oxygen." Anaerobic exercises are exercises that can be performed without additional oxygen consumption. They are shorter bursts of activity that can build strength, increase flexibility, and improve muscle tone and coordination. Both aerobic and anaerobic exercises can increase relaxation and mental well-being.

Aerobic exercise is generally considered the more beneficial for people with diabetes because it lowers blood glucose, increases weight reduction, and improves cardiovascular function. But anaerobic exercise can also be beneficial in controlling diabetes.

Exercises such as stretching, yoga, tai chi, and others have their place in a well-rounded exercise regimen.

Some exercises can be aerobic or anaerobic depending on how they are performed. For example, light weight training performed at a fast pace with increased repetitions and duration can be aerobic. The use of heavier weights with decreased repetitions and duration is considered anaerobic activity.

Regardless of the exercise routine you choose, it is very important to warm up and cool down adequately. A five to ten minute warmup will help your body adjust to the rigors of the main exercise period, and it will help prevent exercise-related injuries and problems. A good warmup should include a variety of stretches and a few minutes of gradually increasing, low-intensity activity. After the main exercise period, a five-minute cool-down will help your body readjust. During the cool-down period, the main exercise activity should be decreased gradually until it becomes low intensity. Light stretching at the end of exercise reduces soreness and increases flexibility.

Strength Training

Strength training, which is usually an anaerobic activity, has enjoyed widespread popularity in recent years. What is strength training? Any exercise that makes muscles work against some kind of resistance, such as weightlifting, pushups, and pull-ups.

Why are so many people adopting strength training programs? Strength training is one of the most effective means of slowing the aging process. Much of the physical decline that people experience as they get older—slowed metabolic rate, obesity, bone loss, weakness, and glucose intolerance—is directly related to loss of muscle mass. And strength training is the most effective type of exercise you can do to build and maintain muscle mass. Here are some specific benefits you can expect from following a forty-five minute strength training program three times a week:

• Your bones will become stronger and denser, and therefore less likely to fracture. Your risk of osteoporosis will greatly decline.

• As you build muscle mass, your metabolic rate will increase, causing you to burn more calories. This, in turn, will make it easier to lose body fat.

- Your body will become firmer and denser. As you gain muscle and lose fat, you may notice that your clothes are looser fitting, even though your weight has not changed. This is because muscle weighs more than fat. If your primary goal is weight loss, don't get discouraged if you are not losing weight as fast as you think you should. Let your appearance be your guide. The best way to monitor your results is to track changes in your body measurements or in your percentage of body fat.

- Tendons and joints become stronger and more elastic, enabling you to perform all activities with less risk of injury.

- Muscles become more sensitive to insulin, which helps reduce blood sugar levels, and improves cholesterol and triglycerides.

Despite all the positive effects of strength training, health professionals have historically advised against weightlifting for people with diabetes. Why? Lifting heavy weights can exacerbate some complications of diabetes such as eye damage, kidney damage, and hypertension. However, researchers are beginning to discover that a moderate type of weightlifting known as *circuit weight training* may be beneficial for some people with diabetes. A circuit may include eight to fifteen resistance exercise stations, each of which works a different muscle group. At each station, you lift a moderate amount of weight for fifteen to twenty repetitions. Then you rest for fifteen to thirty seconds before moving to the next exercise station.

Other examples of light to moderate weight training activities are body toning exercises using free weights or exercise rubber bands. These activities are an especially good place for beginners to start.

Be sure to check with your physician before you begin a circuit training program or any other light to moderate weight training activities. Although not as strenuous as heavy weightlifting, these activities are not recommended for all people with diabetes.

Aerobic Exercise

Aerobic exercise involves repetitive contractions of large muscle groups for a long period of time. Fast walking, running, swimming, dancing, step aerobics, and bicycling are examples of aerobic exercise. Doing a variety of exercises will help prevent boredom and enhance your exercise routine. Exercise should be fun. When exercise is enjoyable, people tend to stick with it.

Walking

Walking is an excellent way to get started with aerobic exercise. It's easy to do and it doesn't take any special equipment. All you need are a good pair of shoes and some good cotton socks, and you can walk in nearly any area. You might try to find someone to walk with you. Walking with someone else can make exercising more enjoyable, and it's safer than walking alone. In addition, if you are accountable to a walking partner, you are more likely to stick with your exercise program.

Additional Aerobic Activities

There are many aerobic activities, which you might not consider exercise, that can lower your blood sugar and burn extra calories. The latest advice for people who don't have time for planned exercise is that they be active at various times throughout the day. For instance, climbing stairs, dancing, doing yard work, vacuuming, and other comparable activities raise your activity level and can improve your blood glucose control. Walk to work, park your car in a parking space farthest from the entrance to the mall, use a push mower instead of a riding mower—you get the picture. Get moving! Instead of watching television or going to the movies during your spare time, take up golf, tennis, volleyball, hiking, or other activities that will get your body going. Table 4.1 will give you some idea of how effectively different activities burn calories and fat.

Armchair Exercises. If you are unable to walk or do other exercises due to conditions such as arthritis, blood vessel disease, or nerve

Table 4.1. Activities That Burn 150 Calories

Activity	Time Required to Expend 150 Calories
SPORTS ACTIVITIES	
Aerobic Dancing (moderate intensity)	21 minutes
Aerobic Dancing (high intensity)	16 minutes
Ballroom Dancing	43 minutes
Basketball	16 minutes
Biking (10 miles per hour)	22 minutes
Canoeing (leisure)	50 minutes
Canoeing (racing)	21 minutes
Golf (putting clubs)	26 minutes
Jumping rope (70 per minute)	14 minutes
Racquetball	13 minutes
Running (9-minute miles)	11 minutes
Running (6-minute miles)	9 minutes
Scuba diving	11 minutes
Swimming (breast stroke)	14 minutes
Tennis (singles)	20 minutes
Volleyball	44 minutes
Walking	27 minutes
Weightlifting (circuit training)	26 minutes
HOUSEWORK	
Mopping	36 minutes
Scrubbing	20 minutes
Vacuuming	48 minutes
Cleaning windows	38 minutes

disease, you should ask your doctor if armchair exercises would be right for you. Armchair exercises, which can be aerobic as well as anaerobic, are becoming increasingly popular among people whose physical activities are restricted for medical reasons. Sources for armchair exercise videos are listed in the back of this book.

GETTING STARTED ON AN EXERCISE PROGRAM

Before you begin an exercise program, it is important that you have a complete physical to make sure that exercising is safe for you. If you have any complications related to diabetes, certain exercises may be potentially dangerous. Be sure to discuss your exercise plan with your doctor.

Target Heart Rate

When you exercise aerobically, your aim is to raise your heart rate to a level that will give you the best and safest results. Therefore, you should aim toward a pre-determined heart rate, or target heart rate. Naturally, you will want to discuss this with your doctor. But you can get an idea of a beneficial target heart rate for people of your age group by subtracting your age from 220 and multiplying your answer by .60 and then by .75. For example, if you are sixty years old, you would do the following arithmetic:

220 minus 60 = 160 = your maximum safe heart rate.
Next multiply: *160 x .60 = 96*
Then multiply: *160 x .75 = 120*

The target heart rate range during exercise for a sixty-year-old is between 96 and 120 beats per minute. For people with diabetes who have heart disease or other complications, the target heart rate may have to be lower.

   Your doctor or diabetes educator can teach you how to check your pulse so that you can monitor your heart rate during exercise. It is important to remember that the above formula may not be appropriate for everyone. Other factors should also be taken into account when determining target heart rate during exercise. You and your physician must consider additional factors such as the presence of heart disease or other physical conditions, which medications you are taking, and your fitness level.

It is important to begin exercising slowly and build up the amount of time and intensity of your activity. How much exercise is enough? Start by doing five to ten minutes of mild to moderate exercise, and build up your endurance and intensity slowly over several weeks and months. For improvement in blood sugar control, exercising at least every other day for twenty to sixty minutes per session is recommended. If you are trying to lose weight, exercise at least thirty to forty-five minutes, five days a week. To maximize health and longevity, the United States Surgeon General recommends that everyone exercise enough to burn at least 150 extra calories per day, or about 1,000 extra calories per week. Table 4.1 presents a number of activities that will help you do just that.

Remember that it is important to select activities that are right for you. Consider the types of activities you enjoy, your present physical condition, and any barriers to exercising that you may have. Lack of time is often given as a reason for not sticking with a program of regular exercise. Look at your schedule and determine the best times to schedule twenty to thirty minutes of exercise. It is important to make exercise a priority in your daily routine!

Safety Considerations During Exercise

No matter what type of exercise you are doing, you must take precautions so that you don't injure yourself or overwork your body. First and foremost, your breathing should be comfortable and regular enough for you to carry on a conversation as you exercise. If you become short of breath or have any pain, stop immediately. Inform your doctor about any chest or leg pain at once. Always take time to warm up before you begin and cool down when you have finished your exercise routine. And always drink plenty of water before, during, and after exercise.

Furthermore, if your blood sugar is above 240 mg/dl and you have ketones in your urine before exercising, delay exercise. If your blood sugar is this high, exercise can cause your blood sugar and ketones levels to rise even higher! There are additional precautions that you should take, which will be discussed in the following sections.

Monitor Your Blood Glucose

It is important that you monitor your blood glucose before and after exercise, and sometimes during exercise when it is of long duration. Anyone who takes diabetes medication is at risk for low blood sugar during exercise. If you do not take medication to control your diabetes, there is no need to increase your food intake before, during, or after exercise. In fact, eating extra food when you don't need it will wipe out the weight-loss benefits of exercise.

Take Extra Precautions if You Take Medication

If you take diabetes medication on a regular basis and your blood sugar is less than 100 mg/dl before exercising, you should have a snack. For longer periods of exercise, you should check your blood glucose and take a snack containing approximately fifteen grams of carbohydrates for every thirty to forty-five minutes of continuous exercise.

If you take insulin on a regular basis, talk to your doctor or diabetes educator and ask for recommendations on how to decrease your insulin or increase your calories to compensate for the blood glucose-lowering effects of exercise. In general, the safest time to exercise for a person who takes diabetes medication is about one to one and a half hours after a meal.

Anyone who takes diabetes medication may be at risk for low blood sugar during or after exercise. If you take diabetes medication, carry something with you that contains real sugar when you exercise. Glucose tablets or hard candies are easy to carry and usually work well to raise your blood sugar if it drops too low. The blood glucose-lowering effects of exercise may last for several hours following the completion of exercise. People who take diabetes pills or insulin are at risk for a condition called *post-exercise late-onset hypoglycemia*. Remember that low blood sugar reactions may occur several hours after exercise is completed. If you take insulin, you may want to ask your doctor about prescribing a glucagon emergency kit. A friend or family member should be taught how to use it in case you have a low blood sugar reaction and cannot help yourself. The inset "Emergency Instructions for Administering Glucagon" in Chapter 5 provides complete instructions for administering glucagon.

Carry Identification

Keep diabetes identification with you when you exercise so that if you are in a situation in which you cannot help yourself, you will be more likely to receive the proper assistance. Wallet cards and jewelry are available in most pharmacies or they can be ordered through the mail.

General Precautions

Performing exercises that involve jarring, such as jogging or trampoline jumping, or that cause straining can be dangerous for people with certain complications of diabetes. Jarring or straining during exercise can increase pressure in small blood vessels. Lifting weights that are too heavy can make blood pressure rise too high in people with hypertension. Be sure to get the go-ahead from your doctor before beginning these activities.

The following precautions should be taken by anyone who exercises:

- Wear cotton socks and shoes that fit well when you exercise. Check your feet before and after exercise to be sure that you don't have blisters, cuts, or any developing problems.

- Avoid intense exercise in extremely hot or cold weather. Avoid exercising in high humidity.

- Before, during, and after exercise, drink plenty of water or fluids that don't contain sugar.

- Stop exercising immediately if you experience any pain or shortness of breath, or if you feel dizzy or faint. Then seek medical attention.

CONCLUSION

Exercise can and should be part of your everyday life, for it is one of the single most effective treatments available for diabetes. Remember to plan your program well, consult with your doctor, and start slowly. By incorporating regular exercise into your life, you will feel better and you will be healthier and happier.

CHAPTER FIVE

Mastering Diabetes Medications

A lthough an excellent diet and regular exercise are essential to your good health, it must be noted that there may be times when your doctor must prescribe medication to bring your blood sugar levels under control. It will help you to know in advance when these medications may be prescribed, what sorts of medications you may need, and how they can help your medical condition. This chapter will discuss the different diabetes medications, medication interactions and precautions, and the effects that many prescription and over-the-counter medications have on diabetes. In addition, there is important information about mixing and injecting various types of insulin.

WHEN IS MEDICATION PRESCRIBED?

It is not unusual for people whose blood sugar is normally controlled without insulin to need diabetes medication from time to time, especially during periods of illness or stress. This is because physical and emotional stressors can cause a release of hormones that oppose the actions of insulin and cause a release of stored glucose. But once their secondary problems have been resolved, most people can discontinue the use of medications, and return to controlling their diabetes with exercise and diet.

WHAT TYPES OF MEDICATION
ARE PRESCRIBED FOR DIABETES?

There are two types of medication prescribed for people with diabetes: oral diabetes medication, which comes in pill form; and insulin, which is injected. Today, there are many new treatment options available that were not available just a few years ago. The availability and versatility of these medications make it possible for you and your doctor to work out a treatment regimen designed specifically for your needs.

ORAL DIABETES MEDICATIONS

Five categories of pills are now available for the treatment of diabetes. Each type of medication works in a different way to improve blood sugar control. Some diabetes pills stimulate the pancreas to produce more insulin, some decrease glucose production by the liver, some help the body use insulin more efficiently, and some slow down the absorption of carbohydrates from the intestines.

Table 5.1 summarizes the different types of oral diabetes medications and presents some important considerations about each type.

Table 5.1. Oral Diabetes Medications

1. CLASS: SULFONYLUREAS

acetohexamide (Dymelor); chlorpropamide (Diabinese); gliclazide; glimepiride (Amaryl); glipizide (Glucotrol, Glucotrol XL); glyburide (Glynase, Diabeta, Micronase); tolazamide (Tolinase); tolbutamide (Orinase)

How They Work

Sulfonylureas work mainly by stimulating the pancreas to produce more insulin. They also improve insulin sensitivity and decrease glucose production in the liver. Sulfonylureas have been used to treat diabetes in the United States for over forty years.

Important Considerations

- Because all sulfonylureas increase insulin secretion, they all have the potential to cause hypoglycemia (low blood sugar).
- Glucotrol is the only diabetes pill that must be taken on an empty stomach, approximately 30 minutes before a meal.

Important Considerations

- Chlorpropamide and Tolinase can interact with alcohol and produce a serious reaction.

- Use of sulfonylureas often results in a weight gain of 5 pounds. This can be especially discouraging for people who are trying to lose weight to help control their diabetes.

- Sulfonylureas can accumulate in the body and cause problems. People who have kidney and liver disease should use them with caution. Chlorpropamide has the longest duration of action—up to 72 hours.

- Rashes and other signs of allergic reactions may occur with use of these medications. Report any signs of allergic reactions to your doctor.

2. CLASS: BIGUANIDE

metformin (Glucophage)

How It Works

Metformin decreases glucose production by the liver. It also improves insulin action and slows absorption of glucose from the small intestines. This medication has been used in some countries for over thirty years.

Important Considerations

- Metformin may cause diarrhea, abdominal bloating, nausea, and vomiting. These problems are ordinarily temporary, and disappear as the body adjusts to the medication. Taking the medication with food, and gradually increasing the amount taken until the target dose is reached, can minimize problems.

- This medication should be used with caution in people with heart disease.

- Metformin should not be used before undergoing medical procedures that use contrast dyes.

- This medication has the potential to cause a rare but serious problem called lactic acidosis. People who have liver or kidney problems should not take this drug because they are more prone to develop this problem. Symptoms of lactic acidosis include weakness, tiredness, muscle pain, trouble breathing, coldness, dizziness, and irregular heartbeat.

- Excessive amounts of alcohol should be avoided when taking metformin. Discuss alcohol use with your doctor or diabetes educator.

- Metformin does not promote weight gain. In fact, most people lose weight when starting on the drug.

Important Considerations

- Improvements in cholesterol and triglyceride levels are a frequent benefit of using this medication.

- Low blood sugar (hypoglycemia) is usually not a problem when metformin is taken alone. But when it is taken with sulfonylureas or insulin, metformin has the potential to cause low blood sugar.

3. CLASS: ALPHA-GLUCOSIDASE INHIBITORS

acarbose (Precose, Prandase); miglitol (Glyset)

How They Work

These medications work in the small intestine to slow the digestion of carbohydrates. This results in lower blood sugar levels after eating.

Important Considerations

- Alpha-glucosidase inhibitors may cause mild to moderate gastrointestinal symptoms such as gas and diarrhea. These problems usually disappear in 3 to 4 weeks. People with chronic intestinal or liver problems should not take these medications. Gradually increasing the dose until the target dose is reached can minimize gastrointestinal problems.

- These medications must be taken with the first bite of each meal.

- These medications do not have a direct effect on fasting blood sugar levels.

- These medications may cause a reduction in triglyceride levels and weight loss.

- These medications taken alone will not cause hypoglycemia, but if they are taken with other diabetes drugs, low blood sugar can result. Alpha-glucosidase inhibitors slow the absorption of some carbohydrates, including table sugar (sucrose); thus, hypoglycemia should be treated with milk, which contains a sugar called lactose, or with glucose tablets.

4. CLASS: THIAZOLIDINEDIONE

troglitazone (Rezulin)

How It Works

This drug decreases insulin resistance, making the body more sensitive to the effects of insulin. It also increases the removal from the bloodstream, and decreases glucose output by the liver.

Important Considerations

- When troglitazone is used with insulin or diabetes pills, the dose must be adjusted based on blood sugar values. Blood sugar monitoring is essential for anyone taking this medication. It takes up to 4 weeks for troglitazone to start lowering blood glucose levels.

- Troglitazone can decrease the effectiveness of birth control pills.

- Troglitazone should be taken once daily with the heaviest meal of the day.

- Troglitazone has the potential to improve cholesterol and triglyceride levels.

- The drug should be used with extreme caution in people with liver and heart disease. Liver tests should be done on all patients before they take troglitazone and, periodically, after they start taking it. Jaundice, nausea, vomiting, abdominal pain, fatigue, dark urine, or any other problem should be reported immediately to your doctor.

5. CLASS: MEGLITINIDE

repaglinide (Prandin)

How It Works

This medication works quickly and for a short time to control rises in blood sugar levels after meals. It stimulates the beta cells in the pancreas to make more insulin.

Important Considerations

- Repaglinide must be taken at the correct time, with meals, to control blood glucose effectively.

- This medication is useful for people who skip meals or delay mealtimes, since it is taken with the meal to boost short-term insulin production.

- This medication can cause hypoglycemia.

- This drug slightly increases the risk of cardiovascular problems when compared with other diabetes pills.

- Sinus and respiratory problems may occur as a side effect of this medication.

- Antibacterial drugs, antifungal drugs, and troglitazone (Rezulin) can interact with this medication.

Remember that diabetes pills are not insulin—insulin cannot be given in pill form to lower blood glucose. Furthermore, diabetes medication should not be used in place of nutrition and exercise therapy in controlling diabetes.

Women with diabetes who are planning pregnancy and cannot control their blood sugar with diet and exercise alone should consult with their physician and start managing their diabetes with insulin *before* becoming pregnant. Diabetes pills should *never* be taken during pregnancy.

Side Effects of Oral Diabetes Medications

All medications have the potential to cause problems and to interact with other medications. Ask your doctor about possible side effects and drug interactions associated with each medication prescribed for you. You can also use Table 5.1 as a general reference. It is imperative that you take the correct dose prescribed by your doctor, that you take your medication at the times indicated, and that you know when and what to report to your doctor. Never change your medication or the amount of medication without your doctor's advice.

INSULIN INJECTIONS

Most people with diabetes fear the possibility of having to take insulin shots. Unfortunately, at present, insulin must be taken by injection or by pump in order to bring blood sugar levels down. Nevertheless, most people who take insulin report that the anticipation of taking insulin shots is much worse than actually taking the shots. The needles manufactured today are much finer than the needles used in the past. They are extremely fine and virtually painless.

Sources of Insulin

There are several different sources of insulin, which may be used alone or in combination with other insulin or oral diabetes medications. Human insulin, beef insulin, and pork insulin are the three different species of insulin available today.

How Does an Insulin Pump Work?

Insulin pumps are small devices that are worn continuously. The pump, which looks somewhat like a pager, contains a small reservoir of insulin. Insulin is "pumped" into the body at a slow, continuous rate through a catheter, or needle, that extends from the device and is inserted into the abdomen. Before meals, a bolus dose of insulin is given to keep post-meal blood sugar levels in check. If the pump is removed for more than a short period of time, insulin shots must be resumed. The insulin pump is not appropriate for everyone. People who use them must have advanced skills in dealing with diabetes and its complications, and must be willing to monitor their blood glucose levels frequently. They also must have good support from their health-care team.

Human insulin does not come from humans, but is manufactured in a laboratory to match insulin produced by the human body. It is used more often than beef or pork insulin, and it is considered better because it is absorbed faster, has a shorter duration of action, and is more predictable. The insulin given before a meal should start working, peak, and begin to wear off while the blood sugar rises, peaks, and goes down after eating. In addition, human insulin is usually less expensive than beef or pork insulin, and produces fewer allergic reactions. People who are opposed to the use of insulin from animal sources may use human insulin. Some people who have used other types of insulin have had difficulty changing to human insulin. Be aware that changing the type of insulin you take can affect your diabetes control. Do not change insulin types without the advice of your doctor.

Types of Insulin

There are several different types of insulin available. Each type of insulin works differently so that the *onset of action, peak of action,* and *duration of action* vary with each one. Onset of action refers to the length of time the injected insulin takes to start working; peak of action refers to the time during which the injected insulin is working at its strongest; and duration of action refers to the length of time the insulin works in the body. Table 5.2 reviews the different types of insulin and how they work in your body. In addition, keep in mind that the injection site, technique of injection, absorption rate, and the individual's body composition and response all have an influence on the onset, peak, and duration of insulin action.

Table 5.2. Comparing Insulin Actions

Insulin Name	Onset of Action	Peak of Action	Duration of Action
Rapid-Acting/ Fastest-Acting (Humalog, lispro)	0–15 minutes	About 60 minutes	Under 5 hours
Short-Acting Insulin (Regular, Humulin R, Novolin R, & others)	30–60 minutes	2–4 hours	6–8 hours
Intermediate-Acting Insulin (NPH, Lente, Humulin N, Novolin N, & others)	1–3 hours	6–10 hours	10–16 hours
Long-Acting Insulin (Ultralente, Humulin U)	4–6 hours	18 hours	24–36 hours

Sliding Scale Insulin

Sliding scale insulin is a supplemental dose of insulin that is given based on blood glucose results. Sliding scale rapid-acting insulin or short-acting insulin is often prescribed when a person with diabetes is ill, or during periods when blood glucose is not under good control. If your doctor prescribes sliding scale insulin, he or she will tell you when to check your blood sugar and take your insulin. It is very important to follow directions precisely. Table 5.3

shows a typical sliding scale. However, do *not* attempt to use the guidelines provided in Table 5.3 on your own, as everyone's response to insulin is different. Your doctor will prescribe sliding scale insulin on an individual basis if needed.

Table 5.3. Using Sliding Scale Insulin

If your premeal blood glucose is:	Take:
150–200 mg/dl	2 units of Humalog insulin
201–250 mg/dl	4 units of Humalog insulin
251–300	6 units of Humalog insulin
Over 300	Take 8 units of Humalog insulin and call the doctor immediately

Side Effects of Insulin

The main problem associated with insulin use is *hypoglycemia*, or low blood sugar. This problem is discussed in detail in Chapter 6. In addition, the inset on page 78 explains how you can use a medication called glucagon to quickly raise your blood sugar level in an emergency. For the most part, though, if you take medication at regular times and plan your meals in conjunction with insulin action, you can decrease the risk of developing hypoglycemia. It is also important to take the correct amount of insulin and diabetes medication to prevent problems with low blood sugar.

Local reactions to insulin are rare, but may occur occasionally. They include itching, redness, and pain at the site of injection. The irritations usually clear up on their own, but should be reported immediately to your doctor. Sometimes antihistamines can ease symptoms. Very rarely, generalized allergic reactions may occur. The use of human insulin can help prevent both localized and generalized allergic reactions. Thickening of the skin or dimpling at injection sites can also occur. Problems can be decreased by using appropriate injection techniques and by rotating injection sites. Any problems related to insulin administration should be discussed with your doctor or diabetes educator.

Emergency Instructions for Administering Glucagon

Glucagon is an emergency medication that raises blood glucose. If you develop hypoglycemia and can't swallow or become unconscious, an injection of glucagon can quickly raise your blood sugar. Friends, family members, co-workers, and other people who are frequently in your company should learn how to help you in the case of an emergency. In particular, they should be taught how to use glucagon in case you are not able to help yourself. Show them how to use glucagon, and let them practice giving you a shot by letting them draw up and administer your insulin from time to time. Glucagon is a safe prescription drug. Because the dose comes premeasured in a kit, there is no danger of overdosing. It should be stored in a place that is easy to get to, and everyone should know where it is kept. Check the expiration dates on your glucagon periodically to ensure that it will work if needed. Follow the instructions below for administering glucagon:

1. *Call 911 or a local emergency number whenever a person with diabetes becomes unconscious. Administer the glucagon while waiting for help to arrive.*

2. *Flip the cap off the bottle of glucagon powder and wipe the top with an alcohol swab.*

3. *Inject all the solution provided into the bottle of glucagon powder.*

4. *Remove the syringe from the bottle and shake it gently until the solution is clear.*

5. *The glucagon should be completely dissolved and look like water. Inject the glucagon immediately after mixing. Glucagon cannot be stored after having been mixed. Inject all the glucagon using the same technique used to inject insulin. (See page 86.)*

6. *Turn the person on his side to prevent choking in case he vomits. The person should wake up in fifteen minutes or less. Feed him as soon as he awakens and can swallow. If he does not awaken after fifteen minutes, another dose can be administered.*

7. *Once the person has awakened and the immediate emergency is over, he should notify his physician about the incident at once so that adjustments can be made and future hypoglycemic reactions can be prevented.*

Many people with diabetes who use insulin will never experience a hypoglycemic episode that requires the use of glucagon. Nevertheless, it is important for family, friends, and others to be prepared to deal with the situation. (See Chapter 6 for information about how to avoid things that precipitate hypoglycemia and how to identify early symptoms of hypoglycemia.)

Insulin and Meal Timing

It is important to note that insulin works in conjunction with food. Your injections should be timed so that your insulin has already begun to work by the time your blood sugar starts to rise after eating. For example, short-acting insulin starts working about thirty minutes after injecting, so it should be taken about thirty minutes before eating. Rapid-acting Humalog insulin, however, may be injected right before eating, because it starts working almost immediately. If you don't eat regular meals, you should talk to your doctor about optional insulin regimens to accommodate your meal patterns. Some people need a snack when their insulin is peaking in their body. If you take insulin at night, you should have a bedtime snack as part of your meal plan.

Prescribed Dosage

Insulin, which is measured in divisions called units, is available in different concentrations. The most commonly prescribed concentration is one hundred units per milliliter, or U-100. The strongest concentration available is 500 units per milliliter, or U-500. Weaker concentrations can also be formulated. Less-concentrated insulin is most often used when insulin is administered to infants. Different types of insulin are available in different countries, so be especially careful when traveling. (See Chapter 8 for more information concerning travel.) The main thing to remember is that there are different types and strengths of insulin. Always check your insulin to be sure you are taking the right kind in the correct amount.

Everyone responds to insulin differently, so some people may be able to control their blood sugar by taking just one shot a day, and others may have to take two or more shots a day. Your doctor will probably have to adjust your insulin several times throughout your lifetime, because your blood sugar levels usually fluctuate depending on your circumstances. Whenever your blood sugar is consistently out of control, the amount of insulin you need changes. Your doctor or diabetes educator can teach you how to adjust insulin on your own. Be aware that adjusting insulin or any medication without your doctor's instruction can be very dangerous!

Drawing Up a Single Type of Insulin

Naturally, you will receive first-hand instructions from your doctor or diabetes educator about the injection of insulin. In addition, you can use the following list as a reference:

1. Wash your hands with soap and water.

2. Take your insulin out of the refrigerator and let it warm to room temperature. Cold insulin stings and is more slowly absorbed than room-temperature insulin. (But never *heat* insulin.)

3. Be sure that you have the right type and concentration of insulin. Check the bottle for cracks or leaks. Always check the expiration date on the label. Short-acting insulin and rapid-acting insulin should always be clear. Other insulins look cloudy (like skim milk). Clumping of particles in the insulin bottle, clouding of clear insulin, discoloration of insulin, or frosting on the glass indicates that the insulin has been chemi-

How to Store Insulin Properly

Insulin may be stored at room temperature, but it will lose its potency sooner if it isn't kept refrigerated. As a general rule, if you use all your insulin within thirty days, you can store it at room temperature. But it's best to store insulin in the refrigerator door or in a cool place, away from heat, direct sunlight, or freezing temperatures.

Insulin syringes can be pre-filled and stored in the refrigerator for up to twenty-one days. They should be stored in a vertical position, preferably with the needles pointing up. If the syringes contain different types of insulin, they should be gently rolled between your palms in order to mix them up before injecting. Pre-filled syringes may also be purchased from a pharmacy. Insulin pens that enable you to "dial a dose" are also available, but they require special training for correct use.

Some people with diabetes use jet injectors instead of needles. The insulin is injected through a very fine stream that pierces the skin. Although these devices may be beneficial for some people, they are not always considered an option, because incorrect use can cause tissue scarring. In addition, they are more expensive than syringes, and special training is needed for people who use these devices.

cally altered and should not be used. Discard any insulin that doesn't look right, or return it to your pharmacy.

4. Get your equipment together. You will need an insulin syringe and an alcohol swab, or alcohol and cotton balls. Draw up your insulin in a clean area.

5. Gently roll cloudy insulin between your hands ten to twenty times to mix it well. Don't shake your insulin; it creates air bubbles.

6. Flip the plastic cap off the top of a new bottle of insulin. Clean the bottle top with an alcohol swab, and allow the top to dry

before you withdraw the insulin. There is no need to save the plastic cap; the rubber stopper will seal the bottle.

7. Pull back on the plunger of the syringe and draw air into it. The amount of air you draw into the syringe should be equal to the amount of insulin you are taking from the bottle. This equalizes pressure inside the bottle and makes it easier to withdraw the insulin.

8. Take the cap off the needle and insert the needle into the insulin bottle through the rubber stopper. Push down on the plunger and inject all the air into the bottle.

9. Leaving the needle in, turn the bottle upside down and slowly draw back the plunger to the desired dose. The end of the plunger should be exactly on the mark for your dose. Precision is important—if your measurement is just one unit off, it can cause big problems for you.

10. Look for air bubbles. If there are air bubbles in your insulin, point the needle upward and gently tap on the syringe over the bubbles until they float to the top; then inject the air back into the insulin bottle and draw the plunger back to your dose. Some bubbles are difficult to get out—if you can't tap them out, push the plunger all the way back in and slowly withdraw the insulin again. The air bubble itself won't hurt you, but it takes up space that insulin would normally fill and causes the dose to be reduced.

11. Recap the needle if it will be a while before you inject yourself. To keep the needle sterile, avoid touching it to anything.

Withdrawing and injecting insulin usually feels awkward at first. This is normal. Be patient with yourself. If you make a mistake, simply start over. Your skill will improve with time and experience.

Mixing Different Types of Insulin

Different types of insulin may be mixed in the same syringe, or they may be bought premixed. Probably the most commonly used premixed insulin is 70 percent intermediate-acting insulin and 30

About Syringes

Insulin syringes are available in different sizes. The largest insulin syringes hold up to 100 units, or one milliliter, of insulin. There are also low-dose syringes available that hold twenty-five, thirty, or fifty units of insulin. Many people prefer them because they are easier to handle and the unit marks are easy to see. A word of warning: be sure to check the markings on the syringes you use. Some syringes have a mark for each unit, and other syringes have a mark for every two units. In addition, the syringe should be marked with the concentration of insulin that is used with it.

It is best not to reuse syringes. Reusing syringes increases the risk of infection at the injection site. Furthermore, reusing a needle will dull the point. Sharp needles make injections more comfortable; so shots with dull needles usually hurt more because they don't pierce the skin as easily as sharp needles. If you must reuse a syringe, replace the cap after injecting. Be careful not to touch anything with the needle, and try to reuse the syringe on the same day. There is no need to wipe needles with alcohol before reusing. The used syringe may be stored at room temperature.

Used syringes and lancets should be disposed of according to local laws. Remember that they are considered biohazardous waste, and they should be disposed of as such. At very least, they should be disposed of in a puncture-proof container, sealed, and marked as biohazardous waste. Containers made for this purpose are available in most pharmacies. Do not recap needles before disposing of them. Do not break needles off or bend them back. Instead, if you must remove the needle, use a needle-clipping device, which you will find in your pharmacy. And remember that you should never put used syringes or needles into your recycle bin. Ask your doctor or diabetes educator about laws concerning biohazardous waste disposal in your area.

percent short-acting insulin. Other premixed combinations are available.

It is often useful to mix different types of insulin together in order to fine-tune blood sugar control. For instance, if you take a mixture of intermediate- and short-acting insulin, the short-acting insulin will start working in thirty minutes to sixty minutes; it will peak in two to four hours; and it will wear off after six to eight hours. Intermediate-acting insulin starts working in one to three hours, reaches its peak between six and ten hours, and lasts for ten to sixteen hours. The actions of the two types of insulin complement each other. As the short-acting insulin wears off, the intermediate-acting insulin begins to peak. You should consult your doctor for information about mixing different types of insulin that are appropriate for your condition.

The following warnings should always be heeded:

- Generally, avoid mixing different brands of insulin.

- NPH and Regular insulin that are mixed together should be used immediately or stored in the refrigerator.

- Do not mix Regular insulin or NPH insulin with lente insulins unless you have been doing this for a while with your doctor's knowledge. However, lente insulin preparations may be mixed together.

- Do not mix any other medication with your insulin.

- Consult the insulin manufacturer or your doctor if you have any questions about mixing insulin.

Drawing Up a Mixed Dose of Insulin

When you withdraw a mixed dose, you can refer to the following list of procedures:

1. Follow the first six steps for drawing up a single injection (page 80). When you get to step 6, clean off the tops of both insulin bottles.

2. Inject air into the bottle of cloudy insulin. The amount of air injected into the bottle of cloudy insulin should be equal the dose of cloudy insulin you will be taking out. Remove the needle from the bottle of cloudy insulin without drawing up the insulin.

3. Inject air into the bottle of clear insulin that is equal to your clear insulin dose. Turn the bottle of clear insulin upside down and withdraw your dose. Remove the needle from the bottle and double-check your dose.

4. Insert the needle back into the bottle of cloudy insulin and pull the plunger back until you add your dose of cloudy insulin to the clear insulin. Be careful at this step—if you draw back too far, you cannot inject insulin back into the bottle. Tap any air bubbles to the top. Be careful not to inject any insulin back into the bottle. Example: Your doctor orders 10 units of NPH insulin and 4 units of Regular insulin. Inject 10 units of air into the NPH insulin bottle without drawing up the insulin. Inject 4 units of air into the Regular insulin bottle and withdraw the insulin. Remove the needle from the bottle and double-check the dose. Next, withdraw 10 units of NPH insulin. Remove the needle from the bottle. The total dose should be 14 units.

5. Remove the needle and get ready for your injection.

Choosing an Injection Site

Insulin may be given in any of the areas illustrated in Figure 5.1. Absorption rates will vary in each injection site, and it is generally recommended that injections be rotated within one area of the body. The abdomen is usually the best site for insulin injections because insulin is absorbed fastest from that area. Some people prefer to do their pre-meal injections in the abdomen and their nighttime injections in the thighs. You should rotate injection sites and space them about one inch apart to avoid over-using one site. Avoid injecting into the two-inch area around your navel, in the groin or inner-thigh area, or near joints, scars, or stretch marks.

If you are planning to exercise, it is not a good idea to inject into areas that you will be exercising. For example, if you are planing to go bicycle riding, don't inject insulin into your thighs. This is because the insulin will be absorbed faster in that area due to the increased circulation during exercise, and you could have problems with hypoglycemia.

Instructions for Injecting Insulin

Again, your doctor or diabetes educator will work with you to give you hands-on experience and instructions for self-injection. The following list can be used for reference:

1. Choose your injection site. Rub it gently to feel for any knots beneath the skin or depressions in the skin. If you find any knots or depressions, do not use that area, and let your doctor know about it.

2. Clean the injection site with an alcohol swab or soap and water. Let it dry completely.

Figure 5.1. Insulin
Injection Sites,
Front of Body

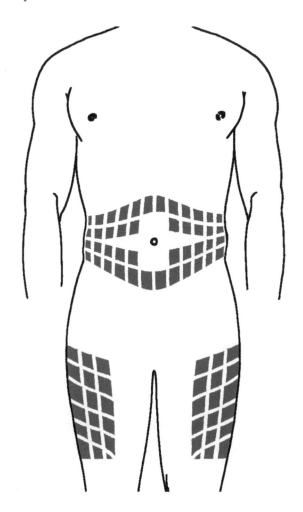

3. Gently pinch up at least one inch of skin with your non-dominant hand.

4. Hold the syringe like a dart in your dominant hand. Quickly push the needle straight into the pinched-up skin at a ninety-degree angle. The hub of the needle should be against the skin. If you are thin, you can insert the needle at a forty-five-degree angle to the skin, or use short needles. Do not insert the needle at an angle that is less than forty-five degrees; if the angle of injection is too shallow, it can cause problems with absorption. Ask your doctor or diabetes educator if short needles would be appropriate for you.

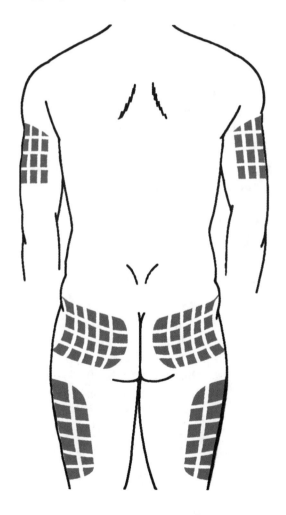

Figure 5.1. Insulin
Injection Sites,
Back of Body

5. Still holding the skin pinched up, push the plunger all the way down to inject the insulin. There is no need to draw back on the plunger.

6. Remove the needle once all of the insulin is injected; cover the site with an alcohol pad, and release the pinched-up skin.

7. Do not rub the injection site. If you see blood after withdrawing the needle, simply apply pressure for a few seconds.

8. Dispose of the used syringe in an appropriate container without recapping the needle or trying to bend or break the needle.

HOW DO OTHER MEDICATIONS AFFECT DIABETES CONTROL?

Many drugs affect blood glucose control. Whenever your doctor prescribes a new medication for you or you purchase an over-the-counter medication, be sure to find out how the new medication may affect your diabetes control. Read all medication labels and instructions carefully; and avoid products that contain sugar, alcohol, or *epinephrine*. If you go to several doctors, be sure that each doctor knows all the medications you are taking. Finally, it's a good idea to use one pharmacy so that you and your pharmacist can get to know each other. The following lists of drugs—legal and illegal—can affect your blood glucose control:

Drugs That Tend to Lower Blood Glucose Levels

Alcohol

Allopurinol

Anabolic steroids (Dianabol)

Aspirin

Beta-Blockers

Chloramphenicol (Chloromycetin)

Clofibrate (Atromid-S)

Coumarin (Dicumarol)

Methyldopa (Aldomet)

Monoamine Oxidase (MAO) Inhibitors (Parnate, Nardil, and others)

Propanolol (Inderal)

Sulfa drugs (Bactrim, Septra, and others)

Tagamet

Drugs That Tend to Raise Blood Glucose Levels

Alcohol (chronic use)
Birth control pills
Caffeine
Calcium channel blockers
   (Calan, Cardizem, and
   Procardia)
Cocaine
Cold remedies
Corticosteroids (Cortisone,
   Decadron, prednisone, and
   others)
Decongestants
Diazoxide (Hyperstat,
   Proglycem)
Diet pills
Diuretics (Diuril, Lasix, Dyazide,
   and others)
Epinephrine (Adrenalin)
Estrogen
Glycerol
Lithium
Niacin
Pentamidine
Phenobarbital
Phenytoin (Dilantin)
Propanolol (Inderal)
Protease inhibitors
Rifampin
Syrups and sugary
   medications
Thyroid medication

CONCLUSION

Many people with diabetes live very well without taking medication. But no matter how faithful you are to your diet and exercise program, and despite all your efforts to avoid illness, stress, and fatigue, you may need oral diabetes medication or insulin on occasions during unusual periods in your life. And you may need diabetes medication if your diabetes control deteriorates over time. The most important thing for your health and well-being is good blood glucose control. With knowledge and the implementation of a good diet and exercise program, and with the variety of options available today in medications used to treat diabetes, you and your doctor can work out a program that's just right for you.

CHAPTER SIX

Dealing With High and Low Blood Glucose Levels

W hen you have a disorder such as diabetes, it is vital that you be aware of the effects it can have on your body, particularly in terms of your blood glucose levels. Knowing the warning signs that your blood glucose levels are reaching dangerously high or low levels may save your life. Although the body has a sort of barometer that can warn you when blood sugar levels are too high or too low, you cannot always rely on it. Many people have high and low blood sugar levels without experiencing any warning symptoms. That's why checking your blood sugar regularly is so important! This chapter will discuss the causes, symptoms, and associated problems of *hyperglycemia* and *hypoglycemia*; and it will tell you what to do to help yourself if you are ever in danger.

WHAT IS HYPERGLYCEMIA?

Hyperglycemia is the medical term for high blood glucose. High blood glucose, which can come on gradually or suddenly, can cause both acute and chronic complications. If you ignore hyperglycemia and your blood glucose levels become extremely elevated, it can bring about severe dehydration and imbalances in your body's chemistry. Over a long period of time, hyperglycemia can affect the blood vessels and nerves throughout the body and cause some of the health problems associated with diabetes. The prevention of hyperglycemia and early intervention if it does occur must be priorities for people with diabetes.

Causes of Hyperglycemia

Hyperglycemia is often preventable. Although there are times when you have no control over its causes, it is helpful to be aware of some circumstances that can cause or exacerbate this condition.

• Eating the wrong things or too much of the right things

• Lack of exercise and activity

• Illness, infection, surgery, heart attack, or any type of physical stress

• Pain

• Psychological or emotional stress

• Taking a medication that affects blood sugar control. (See Chapter 5 for information on medications that affect diabetes control.)

Symptoms of Hyperglycemia

Although not everyone has symptoms of hyperglycemia, most people with diabetes experience at least one of the following indications that their blood sugar is reaching high levels:

• Extreme thirst

• Frequent urination (during the day and at night)

• Extreme hunger

• Fatigue

• Weight loss

• Slow healing of wounds

- Frequent infections. Women with diabetes often have problems with vaginal yeast infections and urinary tract infections.

- Dry, itchy skin. Skin infections are more common in people with diabetes.

- Blurry vision

Don't panic if your blood sugar is too high. There is appropriate action that you can take to make sure that it doesn't lead to severe complications.

What to Do About Hyperglycemia

When your blood sugar begins to get out of control, you should start checking it more frequently. If you find that it is consistently over 140 or 150 mg/dl each time you check it before meals, or if it is over 240 mg/dl twice in a row, call your doctor and get instructions on how to handle the problem. In addition, make sure you are taking your medication correctly. In order to lower blood glucose levels effectively, some diabetes medications must be taken before meals, and others must be taken with meals. Be diligent about following your meal plan. Finally, when your blood sugar levels are high, drink plenty of water or fluid that doesn't contain sugar. Do not exercise if your blood sugar is over 240 mg/dl and you have ketones in your urine. Exercising when blood glucose levels are this high can cause an *increase* in both blood glucose and ketone levels.

Many people with diabetes have problems with hyperglycemia in the morning. If you have insulin-treated diabetes, before treating morning hyperglycemia by increasing the amount of insulin given at night, it is important to determine the cause of the problem. One cause of excessively high blood sugar levels in the morning is called the *dawn phenomenon*. During the early morning hours, the body normally secretes hormones that cause blood sugar levels to rise. Some people may secrete more of these hormones, or may be more sensitive to them. These people will have a greater rise in early morning blood sugar levels than others.

Morning hyperglycemia can also be caused by hypoglycemia

in the early morning hours before rising. This is called the *Somogyi effect*, or *rebound hyperglycemia*. If a person with diabetes has low blood sugar levels during the night, the body may react by releasing stored glucose from the liver into the bloodstream to bring blood sugar levels back up into a normal range. This is a rebound reaction. If the body overreacts and releases too much stored glucose, blood glucose levels will rise excessively and cause hyperglycemia.

If hyperglycemia upon rising is caused by the dawn phenomenon described above, the proper treatment is to increase your intermediate-acting insulin dose before dinner or at bedtime. But if the cause of hyperglycemia upon rising is due to rebound hyperglycemia, the appropriate treatment is to *decrease* your intermediate-acting insulin dose before dinner or at bedtime. It is easy to see why it can be dangerous to adjust insulin on your own. If you have problems with blood glucose control, be sure to work with your doctor or diabetes educator when adjusting your diet and/or medication.

Problems Associated With Hyperglycemia

There are acute problems associated with excessively high blood sugar. *Diabetic ketoacidosis*, or DKA, and *hyperglycemic hyperosmolar nonketotic syndrome*, or HHNS, cause dehydration and imbalance in the body's chemistry. They are treatable conditions, but they can be lethal if they are left unattended.

Diabetic Ketoacidosis (DKA)

Diabetic ketoacidosis usually occurs in people with type 1 diabetes, but people with type 2 diabetes can get it, too. It is a condition in which the body chemistry becomes acidic due to the buildup of toxic substances called *ketones* in the bloodstream. How does this happen? When the body doesn't have enough insulin to enable glucose—its main source of energy—to enter the cells, it is forced to use body fat as an energy source. Ketones are by-products of fat breakdown that can accumulate in the bloodstream and spill over into the urine. Diabetic ketoacidosis occurs when the body chemistry becomes acidic because of the buildup of ketones.

It can develop quickly, and it is life threatening. Ask your doctor or diabetes educator for specific recommendations regarding ketone testing.

Symptoms of DKA. There are a number of symptoms that indicate the development of diabetic ketoacidosis. In addition to the symptoms of hyperglycemia described above, watch out for these symptoms:

- Tiredness and weakness

- Nausea or vomiting

- Pain and cramping in the stomach

- Deep and rapid breathing

- A fruity smell on your breath

Whether or not you have any of the above symptoms, call your doctor without delay if you have blood glucose results over 240 mg/dl and ketones in your urine. If left untreated, DKA can lead to death. If you cannot get in touch with your doctor, go to the nearest hospital emergency room. When your talk to your doctor, have your blood glucose and urine ketone test results available.

Hyperglycemic Hyperosmolar Nonketotic Syndrome (HHNS)

People with type 2 diabetes are more likely to come down with a condition called *hyperglycemic hyperosmolar nonketotic syndrome* (HHNS), or *hyperosmolar coma*. The illness is often confused with other illnesses, and its symptoms may go on for several days without being recognized. HHNS is just as dangerous as diabetic ketoacidosis, but it is different in that ketones are not present in the body; or if they are present, there are only small amounts. People with type 2 diabetes do make insulin, so some glucose can be removed from the bloodstream and used for energy. This prevents significant breakdown of fat for energy and the subsequent formation of ketones. HHNS can be caused by inadequate treatment of diabetes, inadequate fluid intake, loss of large amounts of fluid, infections, heart attack, and other stressors.

Symptoms of HHNS. The symptoms of HHNS are similar to those of diabetic ketoacidosis, except that there are usually fewer stomach problems associated with HHNS. Diabetic ketoacidosis ordinarily comes on suddenly, whereas HHNS generally develops gradually. If ketones are present, there are only small amounts. Dehydration is usually more severe with HHNS than with DKA, and the mortality rate is higher. Because of severe dehydration, a person with HHNS may experience confusion and other neurological changes. This condition may produce mental changes that are similar to those experienced by stroke victims. The symptoms should go away when the person is rehydrated and blood chemistry gets back to normal.

What to Do About DKA and HHNS

DKA and HHNS are treated almost identically. Patients are given fluids for rehydration and insulin to get their blood glucose levels down. Then their *electrolytes*—sodium, potassium, and others—are monitored and they are treated for any imbalances in body chemistry. Anyone who falls victim to these conditions should learn about diabetes care to avoid any further problems.

WHAT IS HYPOGLYCEMIA?

The symptoms of hypoglycemia, or low blood sugar, usually occur when blood sugar levels are below 70 mg/dl. This condition is also called *insulin reaction* in people who take insulin. Hypoglycemia occurs more often in people who take insulin, but it can also occur in people who take certain types of diabetes pills. Hypoglycemia usually comes on suddenly, and it is important to treat it immediately. The condition progresses through stages—mild, moderate, and severe. People with severe hypoglycemia can become disoriented, pass out, have seizures, or lapse into a coma. Hypoglycemia can increase the chance of having an accident while driving, cooking, or participating in other potentially dangerous activities.

Over 50 percent of hypoglycemic episodes occur during sleep. For this reason, you are advised to check your blood glucose during the night between 2:00 and 4:00 A.M. once or twice a week. If you take insulin or certain oral diabetes medications, you should eat a bedtime snack in order to avoid hypoglycemia during sleep. This should be considered part of your meal plan, not extra food.

Causes of Hypoglycemia

Hypoglycemia can be brought on by a number of factors. You will see by studying the following list of causes that the condition is often avoidable if you are diligent about taking care of yourself:

- Taking too high a dose of certain diabetes pills or insulin

- Skipping or delaying meals

- Not eating enough food

- Exercising or doing more physical activity than usual—activities such as yard work and housework count! Exercise can lower blood sugar levels for up to twelve to twenty-four hours

- Drinking alcohol can cause low blood sugar. Be sure to eat when you drink alcohol, and check your blood glucose more diligently after drinking alcoholic beverages

- Taking certain over-the-counter and prescription drugs (refer to the list in Chapter 5, page 88)

- Problems with nutrient absorption and gastric emptying in the gastrointestinal tract

In addition, women may experience a change in their hormones at the beginning of their menstrual period, which can result in lower blood sugar. If this happens, you may have to decrease your insulin at the onset of your menstrual flow. Speak with your doctor or diabetes educator if you have fluctuations in your blood sugar levels during your cycle. Women with diabetes who take insulin also have an increased risk of developing hypoglycemia immediately after giving birth. Fluctuating hormone levels during menopause can also cause problems with hypoglycemia in women who take diabetes medication.

Symptoms of Hypoglycemia

Some symptoms of hypoglycemia can easily be confused with those of hyperglycemia. It is also possible to have hypoglycemia without having symptoms. In addition, symptoms may fluctuate from time to time, or they may decrease over time. This makes it all the more important that you check your blood sugar frequently if you have any of symptoms of hypoglycemia. You may have one or more of the following indications that your blood sugar levels are dangerously low:

- Shakiness and nervousness

- Extreme hunger

- Sweating (if you experience hypoglycemia at night, you may wake up with wet sheets)

- Tingling sensations around the mouth

- Rapid heartbeat

- Feeling cold and clammy

- Blurry vision

- Headache

- Dizziness

- Extreme fatigue, weakness, or drowsiness

- Irritability

- Inability to think clearly, confusion

What to Do About Hypoglycemia

If it is not treated promptly, hypoglycemia can cause disorientation, seizures, and loss of consciousness. If you feel that you are developing hypoglycemia, check your blood sugar if you have a monitor available. If you experience any of the symptoms described above, but cannot check your blood sugar, go ahead and treat yourself as if you do have low blood sugar. The following are general recommendations for treating hypoglycemia. Speak with your doctor or diabetes educator to get specific instructions for your particular case.

1. Quickly eat or drink something containing ten to fifteen grams of simple carbohydrate. Choose one of the following: one-half cup of orange or apple juice (do not add sugar to it), one-half cup of regular soft drink, one cup of milk, one tablespoon of sugar or honey, two or three glucose tablets, two tablespoons of raisins, three pieces of hard candy, or another source of quick sugar. Always keep a source of quick sugar on hand—for instance, in your car, purse, or pocket—especially if you are alone.

2. You should feel better in ten or fifteen minutes. Recheck your blood sugar to be sure it is up to normal levels and then eat something with a little protein in it; if it is mealtime, go ahead and eat you meal.

3. If low blood sugar is not corrected in fifteen minutes, repeat the treatment described above.

4. Recheck your blood sugar periodically throughout the day to be sure it is within normal limits.

5. Try to identify the cause of your hypoglycemic episode, and correct it to avoid future problems.

6. Report the problem to your physician and diabetes educator. They can help you make appropriate adjustments.

7. Avoid over-treating hypoglycemia. You want to increase blood sugar values to the normal range, not above normal!

Should you experience severe hypoglycemia, you will need help from others. Your family, friends, and co-workers should know how to help you in the case of emergency. (See the inset in Chapter 5, page 78, "Emergency Instructions for Administering Glucagon.")

Problems Associated With Hypoglycemia

There are some important considerations to bear in mind concerning hypoglycemia. Some people are unable to detect hypoglycemia, or they confuse the symptoms of hypoglycemia with those of hyperglycemia. Checking blood sugar levels when odd feelings are present can help you avoid this pitfall. There is also a condition called *hypoglycemia unawareness* that develops in some people with diabetes. As its name implies, people with this problem fail to detect any symptoms of low blood sugar. The condition can develop over time and is often related to nerve damage from chronically high blood glucose levels. Some people who keep their blood glucose levels in the lower end of the normal range have problems with hypoglycemia unawareness. If you fall into this category, you should keep your blood glucose in the higher end of the normal range. In addition, some drugs can mask the symptoms of hypoglycemia or make it difficult for your body to recover from it. The only sure way to detect hypoglycemia is to monitor your blood sugar on a regular basis or if suspicious symptoms arise.

Some people are so fearful of hypoglycemia that they don't adequately control their blood sugar levels. Having knowledge about the disorder and being prepared to treat it appropriately can help you avoid this dangerous pitfall. Be sure to discuss your particular blood glucose target levels with your doctor and diabetes educator.

CONCLUSION

As you see, hyperglycemia and hypoglycemia are very different from one another in terms of their causes. Their symptoms, however, can be confused. For this reason, it is essential that you check your blood glucose at regular intervals and that you check it more frequently when you notice it is getting out of control and when you feel any abnormal sensation. Both conditions can be prevented or controlled. But remember that if they do develop and are left untreated, they can they can cause damage to the body or they can be deadly.

CHAPTER SEVEN

Preventing Complications

A s you have learned in earlier chapters, over long periods of time, high levels of blood glucose can damage blood vessels and nerves throughout the body. In turn, this can cause diseases of the eyes, kidneys, feet, nervous system, and cardiovascular system. High blood sugar levels also decrease the body's ability to fight infection.

What can be done to prevent the development of diabetes-related complications? The most important measures you can take are to maintain excellent blood sugar control and to take good care of yourself every day. Regular health screenings and checkups are important to prevent complications and to detect any early signs of complications. By staying informed about the long-term complications of diabetes and the most up-to-date recommendations and treatments, you will be better able to make wise decisions concerning your health care. This chapter will review the complications associated with diabetes, and will discuss measures you can take to prevent their development.

HIGH BLOOD PRESSURE

Because high blood pressure can exacerbate diabetes-related complications, the control of blood pressure must be a priority for people with diabetes. Unfortunately, abnormally high blood pressure, also called *hypertension,* is all too common in countries where people's diet and exercise habits leave much to be desired. For instance, one in four American adults has high blood pressure. Canada follows closely, with 22 percent of adults affected. And since high blood pressure may not produce outward symptoms, many people are not even aware that they have it. Don't let the absence of symptoms fool you! The heart must work harder to pump the blood through the cardiovascular system of a hypertensive person, so even a slightly elevated blood pressure can increase the chance of having a heart attack or stroke.

Symptoms of High Blood Pressure

As already mentioned, high blood pressure usually produces no outward symptoms, so many people are unaware that they have it. Generally, this problem is discovered only as the result of a physical examination.

When you have your blood pressure measured, you are actually measuring the force exerted by the blood on the walls of your blood vessels. Two numbers are used to measure this force. The top number, or *systolic blood pressure,* indicates the pressure inside the arteries when the heart contracts. The bottom number, or *diastolic blood pressure,* indicates the pressure inside the arteries when the heart relaxes between beats. What is a normal blood pressure reading? In general, normal is considered to be around 120/80. Readings of 140/90 and above are considered high.

Preventing High Blood Pressure

What can you do about high blood pressure? First, eat foods that are rich in potassium, calcium, and magnesium. These minerals are essential to blood pressure control. At the same time, avoid excess sodium, which causes fluid retention and raises blood pressure. People with type 2 diabetes tend to be more sensitive to sodium than the general population. If you adopt a low-fat, low-salt diet that includes plenty of vegetables, fruits, legumes, whole grains, and calcium-rich foods, you will automatically get the nutrients you need. Second, if you must lose weight, control your calorie intake to allow for gradual weight loss. Losing just ten pounds can significantly reduce blood pressure in many people. This is especially true for people who tend to carry their excess weight around their middle. Third, exercise regularly. This will keep your cardiovascular system strong, encourage weight loss, and help you deal with stress, which is a major cause of high blood pressure. And finally, don't smoke and don't drink excessive amounts of alcohol. These simple measures are so powerful that they can eliminate the need for medication in many people.

ATHEROSCLEROSIS

Atherosclerosis occurs when plaque, which is made up of fat and cholesterol, becomes deposited on the walls of the arteries and, to a lesser extent, the veins. This narrows the blood vessels, and eventually makes them hard and inelastic. If measures are not taken to reverse plaque buildup, the blood vessels can become so narrow that they clog easily, preventing the blood from carrying oxygen and nutrients to body tissues. At this point, the body becomes vulnerable to heart attacks, strokes, and the development of leg and foot problems that can lead to amputation.

Atherosclerosis is a major factor in the development of coronary artery disease, a disorder in which the arteries that supply blood to the heart become blocked with plaque. Although coronary artery disease is a concern for everyone, people with diabetes are two to twelve times more likely to develop heart disease than are people who do not have this disorder. In addition, people with diabetes develop these problems at an earlier age. Some studies show that diseases of the arteries which supply blood to the heart account for over half of all deaths in people with diabetes. And strokes are also more common in people with diabetes. For all these reasons, the prevention and treatment of atherosclerosis is a key element of good diabetes care.

Symptoms of Atherosclerosis

Chest pain and shortness of breath are perhaps the most common signs of all types of heart disease, including atherosclerosis. Such

Understanding Your Blood Cholesterol Level

High blood cholesterol is a strong risk factor in the development of atherosclerosis. Fortunately, the guidelines presented in this book for a healthy low-fat diet can dramatically reduce blood cholesterol levels for most people. Everyone over the age of twenty should have a cholesterol test at least once every five years. This inset explains what blood cholesterol is, and shows you how to interpret your cholesterol test results.

Cholesterol circulates in the bloodstream in particles called lipoproteins. Two kinds of lipoproteins are measured in a blood cholesterol test. Low-density lipoproteins, or LDL, also known as bad cholesterol, transport cholesterol through the bloodstream to

symptoms should always be taken seriously. Other signs of atherosclerotic disease may include painful leg cramps, pain that goes away with rest, dizzy spells, weak spells, indigestion, and the slow healing of wounds. Although the body usually gives warning signs that alert people to the presence of atherosclerosis, sometimes there are no symptoms at all. In fact, people with diabetes can have so-called *silent* heart attacks, which are sometimes associated with diabetes-related nerve damage.

Preventing Atherosclerosis

Measures can be taken to decrease the risk of developing atherosclerotic disease related to diabetes. First, your doctor should monitor your blood glucose, blood pressure, and cholesterol and triglyceride levels. People over the age of thirty-five should also have a *stress electrocardiogram*—an EKG or ECG—before they begin an exercise program.

In addition to regular monitoring by your doctor, it is essential that you do all that you can to prevent the conditions that lead to *the cells of the body. Here, it is made into vitamin D or various hormones, or it may be incorporated into cell membranes. If LDL is loaded down with more cholesterol than the cells can use, the excess collects on artery walls and forms plaque, which can eventually block arteries and cause a heart attack or stroke.*

High-density lipoproteins, or HDL, also known as good cholesterol, carry cholesterol away from the cells and back to the liver for recycling or disposal. As you might guess, the worst case scenario would be to have high LDL cholesterol and low HDL cholesterol. In this situation, lots of cholesterol is being shipped out into the bloodstream, and not enough is being shipped to the liver for disposal, leaving plenty of cholesterol to form plaque in the blood vessels. The following table categorizes levels of total cholesterol, LDL, and HDL in relation to the risk of developing heart disease.

atherosclerosis. What specific measures can you take? Good nutrition and regular exercise can help control blood glucose, cholesterol, and triglyceride levels; help keep blood pressure low; and control weight gain—all of which will help keep blood vessels clear and improve circulation. Regular exercise alone has been shown to reduce the risk of developing heart disease *by up to 50 percent.*

In addition to a healthy diet and an exercise program, it is important that you avoid habits that increase the risk of atherosclerosis. Smoking increases the risk of cardiovascular conditions in all people, but is especially dangerous for people who have diabetes. Insulin resistance is higher in smokers. If you do smoke, quitting would be one of the best things you can do to improve your health and extend your life. Even if you have smoked for years, you can greatly enhance your health by quitting now.

If blood cholesterol and triglyceride levels cannot be reasonably controlled by the lifestyle changes discussed above, your doctor may consider prescribing medication that can help.

Since the ratio of LDL to HDL in your blood determines how

Table 7.1. Cholesterol and Heart Disease Risk in Adults

Fraction Measured	Low Risk	Intermediate Risk	High Risk
Total Cholesterol	Less than 200	200–239	240 and above
LDL Cholesterol	Less than 130	131–159	160 and above
HDL Cholesterol	60 and above	35–59	Less than 35

much cholesterol is available for deposit in blood vessels, your cholesterol test will probably list the LDL/HDL ratio or the total cholesterol/HDL ratio. Ideally, you should have an LDL/HDL ratio of 3 or less—which means that you have no more than 3 times as much bad cholesterol as good cholesterol—and a total cholesterol/HDL ratio of 4.5 or less—which means that you have no more than 4.5 times as much total cholesterol as good cholesterol. Triglycerides should preferably be less than 200 mg/dl.

Dietary changes can dramatically reduce blood cholesterol and reduce your risk of getting atherosclerosis. How? Primarily, by lowering your LDL cholesterol. You can raise your HDL cholesterol mainly by exercising, maintaining a healthy body weight, and giving up smoking.

EYE DISORDERS

Changes in vision may occur in people with diabetes due to changes in refraction related to the fluctuation of blood sugar levels. This is an acute problem that is reversible when blood sugar levels are brought under control. Long-term diabetes is the leading cause of the onset of blindness and loss of vision in adults. *Diabetic retinopathy,* which has the most serious consequences of all diabetes-related eye conditions, is caused by damage to the tiny blood vessels that supply the retina of the eye. This complication develops over time—the longer a person has diabetes, the more likely it is that retinopathy will develop. In addition, the probability of developing diabetic retinopathy is greater in people who have both diabetes and high blood pressure.

Other eye complications that may be related to diabetes include *glaucoma*, a condition in which the pressure inside the eye increases and damages the optic nerve; and *cataracts*, which are opaque particles inside the lens of the eye that cloud vision. People with diabetes are twice as likely to develop glaucoma and cataracts as are people without this disorder. Additional problems can include damage to the nerves that control the eye, and changes in the eye's lens.

Symptoms of Eye Disorders

Many people with diabetes report that blurry vision was one of their first symptoms of diabetes. In fact, vision problems often prompt people with diabetes to seek medical help in the first place. But it is important to remember that over time, high blood sugar levels can damage the eyes without causing any changes in vision. This is why regular examinations and follow-ups with an eye doctor are essential. When eye problems are caught early, much can be done to treat them before permanent damage is done. Most of the conditions described above can be treated with medication, laser surgeries, or other surgeries.

Preventing Eye Disorders

The risk of diabetes-related eye disease can be decreased with proper care. The following suggestions can help you avoid many eye disorders caused by diabetes.

- Keep your blood glucose levels and blood pressure under control.

- If you have type 2 diabetes, schedule an eye exam. This exam should take place six to eight weeks after you get your blood sugar levels under control. It is advisable for all people with type 2 diabetes to have their eyes examined by a qualified physician who specializes in the management of eye disease in people with diabetes. In general, this should be done annually. People with type 1 diabetes should be screened annually beginning five years after the diagnosis of diabetes, and more often if they have known eye problems.

- Regular follow-up is essential. Eye problems can be treated more successfully when they are caught early. Remember that eye problems may occur without warning signs.

- Smoking constricts blood vessels and makes them narrower. It also increases blood pressure, which can make eye problems worse. If you smoke, it's best that you quit—for your eyes and your overall health.

- Call your doctor if you see light flashes, dark spots, or rings around lights, or have any problems with blurry vision.

- Remember that heavy weightlifting and exercises that cause you to strain can worsen existing diabetic eye problems. Jarring exercises and exercises that cause the head to be below the heart can also be dangerous if you have underlying eye problems. Ask your doctor about the safety of any exercise routine.

- Women with diabetes who become pregnant should have an eye exam during the first three months of pregnancy, and should be monitored closely throughout pregnancy. If you are planning to become pregnant, take into account the risk of developing diabetic retinopathy.

KIDNEY DISEASE

The kidneys maintain the body's internal environment by controlling its fluid and electrolyte levels, and by removing its waste products. The kidneys also work along with other organs to control blood pressure and produce red blood cells.

Diabetic nephropathy is the medical term used to describe kidney disease caused by diabetes. The nephrons are the kidneys' filtering units. Diabetic nephropathy occurs when the tiny blood vessels in the nephrons are damaged as a result of high blood pressure and high blood sugar levels, and fail to function effectively. Fluids then build up in the body, throwing the body's chemistry out of balance. In addition, waste products are not entirely eliminated.

Symptoms of Kidney Disease

There are different stages of kidney disease. In the early stages, kidney disease is usually *silent*—there may no outward signs to warn that the kidneys are not functioning properly. However, this is the point at which kidney disease can be treated most effectively. That's why regular visits with your doctor and screenings for early signs of kidney disease are so important.

Preventing Kidney Disease

What measures can you take to prevent kidney disease? The following steps can help you keep your kidneys healthy and functioning well.

- Control your blood glucose and blood pressure. If you have high blood pressure, studies have shown that a category of blood pressure medications called ACE inhibitors are often effective in improving kidney problems and slowing down the progression of kidney disease. Ask your doctor if ACE inhibitors would be beneficial to you.

- See your doctor immediately if you have a bladder or kidney infection. Signs of a urinary tract infection include pain and burning with urination, frequent urination, cloudy or bloody urine, foul-smelling urine, back pain, chills, and fever.

- Be sure that your doctor checks your urine for *microalbuminuria* at least once a year. This is a simple lab test that can be done to catch kidney problems in the earliest stages. Microalbuminuria, an abnormal presence of small amounts of protein in the urine, may indicate early changes in kidney function. If left untreated, this condition can progress to kidney disease. If protein is detected, appropriate changes in treatment can be implemented to prevent problems from worsening. Other blood and urine tests are also available to detect kidney disease and assess kidney function.

- Smoking can worsen kidney problems. If you do smoke, seriously consider quitting!

- If you are at risk for kidney problems or know that you have kidney problems, see a dietitian to be sure you are not getting too much protein in your diet. The amount of protein that you eat can greatly affect kidney function.

- Avoid drugs that are hard on the kidneys whenever possible. People with kidney problems should be monitored carefully if they take aminoglycosides (gentamicin and others), if they take nonsteroidal anti-inflammatory drugs (ibuprofen and others), or if they undergo any procedures in which radiographic dye is used (cardiac catheterization, for example).

- Ask your doctor about the safety of any exercise routine. Excessive increases in blood pressure can damage the kidneys.

FOOT AND LOWER LEG PROBLEMS

Leg and foot problems related to diabetes result from damage to the nerves and blood vessels that supply the legs and feet. Loss of sensation due to nerve damage in the feet is the main cause of foot problems in people with diabetes. If you have a loss of feeling in your feet, you cannot rely on pain to warn you of foot injuries, and problems can go undetected unless you visually examine your feet. Nerve damage can also cause the feet to change shape, increasing the risk of foot problems. To make matters worse, high blood sugar levels and poor circulation slow down the healing process, causing diabetic foot problems to quickly become very serious.

Peripheral vascular disease is an underlying factor in the development of many of the lower leg and foot problems associated with diabetes. This disorder, which is a common complication of diabetes, is caused by atherosclerosis, the buildup of plaque within the blood vessels. As the plaque builds up, blood flow to the lower legs and feet is decreased.

Symptoms of Foot and Lower Leg Problems

A number of symptoms can signal diabetes-related problems of the feet and legs. These include loss of sensation in the legs and feet; leg pain that accompanies exercise, but eases with rest; pain in the legs and feet at night; and chronically cold feet. In addition, the skin of the lower legs and feet may look shiny and hairless. Bruises, sores, and hot, swollen, tender areas of the feet may also be a sign of problems.

Preventing Foot and Lower Leg Problems

Because they have their root in poor circulation and other general complications of diabetes, many foot and leg problems can be avoided by maintaining good blood sugar control through a healthy diet and an appropriate exercise regimen. Other than this, of course, the prevention of problems through proper foot and skin care and early intervention when foot problems do occur are essential aspects of diabetes self-care. Many lower extremity amputations could have been prevented if proper foot care had been practiced or if prompt action had been taken at the first sign of foot problems.

It is vital that you do all you can to protect your feet. Avoid going barefoot, even indoors. Make sure that your shoes fit well; shoes should be comfortable at the time they are purchased. Avoid wearing heels that are too high, and shoes with toes that are pointed or too narrow. Get into the habit of running your hand down into your shoe and feeling for rocks or sharp objects before putting your shoes on. If you swim, it is a good idea to wear water shoes—the bottoms of pools can be rough, and pool tiles or cement often have sharp edges.

Keep the skin on your feet clean, dry, and healthy. Your skin protects your body from bacterial invasion. If your skin cracks, bacteria can enter the body through the break and cause infection. To keep the skin on your feet soft and supple, apply lotion or petroleum jelly to dry skin after your bath or shower. Avoid applying lotion between the toes, though, because this can cause athlete's foot. Soaking your feet can dry out your skin, so avoid soaking unless your physician tells you to do so.

Toenails that are not trimmed properly can press into adjacent toes and cut the skin. Your toenails should be trimmed straight across, and should not be cut too short. If your toenails are thick, you may find that it is easier to trim them after your shower or bath. File away sharp edges with an emery board, not a metal file.

Before bathing, test the bath water with your elbow or a bath thermometer to avoid scalding your feet. Remember that you may not be able to detect high temperatures with your feet if you have nerve damage. For the same reason, you should not use hot water bottles, heating pads, or electric blankets. It is also a good idea to wear clean, absorbent socks to help your feet stay dry and prevent blistering. Also protect yourself from insect bites. Bites from mosquitoes, spiders, ants, and other insects can be disastrous for a person with diabetes.

Never perform "home operations" by cutting corns or calluses. Also avoid using chemical corn, callus, or wart removers. A podiatrist can help you with these problems.

Identify problems early so that swift action can be taken. Look at your feet and examine them thoroughly at least once a day, and also after exercising. Visually examine and feel the top and bottom of your feet, the back of your heels, and the areas around your ankles and between your toes. If you can't see these areas easily, use a hand mirror or have someone help you examine your feet. You should be looking and feeling for cuts, blisters, insect bites, bruises, sores, or any areas that are red, hot, swollen, or tender. Immediately report any problems that you identify to your doctor. In addition, have your doctor check your feet at each visit.

If you are at risk for the development of foot problems, your doctor may prescribe special shoes or insoles. Medicare and most insurance companies will cover at least part of their costs, since they can prevent severe complications and decrease the risk of amputation.

PROBLEMS OF THE AUTONOMIC NERVOUS SYSTEM

Damage to the *autonomic nervous system,* the part of the nervous system that controls involuntary actions such as breathing and digestion, is a well-known complication of diabetes. Nerve injury occurs because diabetes prevents glucose from being metabolized properly and causes blood supply to be inadequate. This damage, which is referred to as *autonomic neuropathy,* can lead to a wide range of conditions affecting systems throughout the body.

Symptoms of Autonomic Nervous System Problems

Because this diabetes complication can affect so many different systems, symptoms can vary. They can involve problems emptying the bladder, sexual dysfunction, heartburn and other gastrointestinal disorders, dizziness, and a variety of other problems.

Types of Autonomic Nervous System Problems

Bladder Problems

Bladder problems resulting from autonomic neuropathy cause an inability to detect when the bladder is full. A person with this problem may not be able to empty the bladder completely. Urinary tract infections may be more frequent due to urine retention. If you have this condition, you should get into the habit of feeling your bladder periodically and attempting to urinate every few hours. Your doctor may prescribe medications to help relieve this condition.

Gastrointestinal Problems

Delayed emptying of the stomach contents after eating is often the underlying cause of gastrointestinal problems in people with diabetes. It is estimated that 40 percent of people with diabetes have *delayed gastric emptying*, the medical term for this condition. This problem causes variances in digestion and food absorption.

Symptoms of upper gastrointestinal problems caused by autonomic neuropathy include feelings of fullness in the stomach after eating, feeling full early when eating, experiencing hypoglycemic episodes after eating, heartburn, abdominal pain and bloating, reflux, vomiting of undigested food, and anorexia. These conditions may be relieved by eating small frequent meals; implementing a low-fiber, low-fat diet; and drinking liquid meals. Your physician may also be able to provide medication that reduces symptom severity.

Neuropathy-related problems of the lower gastrointestinal tract can vary from constipation to diarrhea. Diet therapy and medications are usually prescribed for these conditions.

Heart and Blood Pressure Problems

Autonomic neuropathy can also affect heart rate and blood pressure. The person with autonomic neuropathy may have a fixed heart rate, meaning that the body does not adjust properly to an increased activity level. Or autonomic neuropathy may lead to *orthostatic hypotension,* a problem that causes a drop in blood pressure when you move from a lying-down position to a standing position. If you experience dizziness, lightheadedness, weakness, or vision changes upon rising, remember to always get up slowly. In addition, be sure to avoid strenuous activity. Diet and medication therapy may be used to help with these problems.

Other Problems

Autonomic neuropathy can also affect the body's ability to detect and respond to hypoglycemia, or low blood sugar. Blood glucose monitoring, with higher blood glucose target goals, is imperative for someone with this condition.

Autonomic neuropathy can also impair the body's ability to sweat, increasing the risk of heat stroke and foot problems due to dry feet. The nerves that control the pupils of the eyes may also be affected by this condition, making it difficult for the pupils to adjust to darkness. Driving at night should be avoided.

Preventing Autonomic Nervous System Problems

Because autonomic nervous system problems typically have their root in high blood sugar levels, you can avoid or slow the progression of a good many of the conditions just described by following a proper diet, getting adequate exercise, and going for regular medical checkups.

SKIN PROBLEMS

Your skin is the first line of defense against invasion by germs and the development of subsequent infection. Unfortunately, people with diabetes are more prone to skin infection than are people without this condition This is due both to nerve damage, which can make repeated injury to the skin more likely, and to poor circulation, which can lead to diabetic ulcers and cause all wounds to heal more slowly.

Symptoms of Skin Problems

Because the skin is so visible, skin problems are relatively easy to detect—as long as you keep alert to their occurrence. Sores that do not heal, and redness, swelling, pus, heat, and pain may all signal the presence of an infection. Any of these symptoms should be taken seriously and brought to the attention of your doctor.

Preventing Skin Problems

Although skin problems are a common complication of diabetes, with proper care, problems can usually be avoided. The following measures should help your skin stay healthy and resistant to damage and infection.

- Bathe or shower daily using mild soap.

- Use lukewarm water for bathing. Hot water will dry your skin out and can scald you.

- Use lotion after your bath or shower to keep your skin soft and supple. This will help prevent skin cracks and breaks.

- If you must stay in the sun for long periods of time, use a sunscreen for protection.

- To avoid frostbite, stay indoors in extremely cold weather and dress warmly when you do go out.

- Avoid any injury to the skin. When injury does occur, keep any cuts or sores clean and covered with a bandage.

SEXUAL PROBLEMS

It is estimated that up to 35 percent of women and 75 percent of men with diabetes experience sexual problems related to the effects of the disease. Such problems are often the result of nerve damage and circulation problems, but can also be related to medications, stress, and other factors. Unfortunately, physicians and patients are often hesitant to bring up the subject of sex.

The good news is that various treatments are now offered to

people who have sexual problems. So if you or your partner have a problem with sexual functioning, be sure to speak with your doctor. If you are not comfortable discussing this matter with your doctor, you might consider asking your partner to bring it up. You might also consider finding a doctor with whom you feel comfortable, or you may prefer to see a doctor who specializes in sexual problems. A urologist would be helpful for men with sexual problems, and a gynecologist would be helpful for women with sexual problems.

People with diabetes may feel depressed at times due to their health problems. This depression, too, can affect sexual functioning. Depression that is severe and affects normal daily functioning should be discussed with your doctor promptly so that you can be treated appropriately.

Symptoms of Sexual Problems

Symptoms of diabetes-related sexual problems vary according to gender and to the underlying physical problem. These symptoms may include difficulty in becoming aroused, decreased vaginal lubrication, difficulty in reaching orgasm, chronic vaginal infections, and impotence.

Types of Sexual Problems

Problems Particular to Women

Women who have sexual problems related to diabetes may have difficulty becoming aroused, decreased vaginal lubrication, and fewer orgasms. Any woman who experiences pain during intercourse should be examined by a gynecologist. Vaginal lubricant creams or estrogen creams may improve some of these symptoms.

Women with diabetes have an increased frequency of vaginal yeast infections and other vaginal infections, which can affect health and sexual function. Report frequent vaginal yeast infections to your doctor. Although many over-the-counter preparations are now available to treat yeast infections, you must not treat vaginal infections without telling your doctor about them. Your doctor should be made aware of *any* infections. Symptoms of a vaginal infection may include an odorous vaginal discharge and itching. As with many other complications of diabetes, controlling your blood sugar can decrease the occurrence of vaginal infections.

Problems Particular to Men

Men with sexual problems related to diabetes may have problems getting an erection even though they have a normal sex drive. The medical terms used to describe this condition are *impotence* and *erectile dysfunction*. The underlying cause of erectile dysfunction must be determined by a doctor—generally a urologist, who specializes in erectile dysfunction—before it can be treated effectively. Alcohol and drug use, blood pressure medications, hormone deficiencies, psychological problems, and stress can also add to problems of this nature.

There are a number of treatment options available today to treat erectile dysfunction. Vacuum devices, penile implants, oral medications, injectable medications, medications that are inserted through the urethra, or surgery to correct circulatory problems may be prescribed by doctors.

Retrograde ejaculation is a rare condition caused by damage to the nerves that coordinate the sequence of ejaculation. This disorder causes semen to back up into the bladder instead of being ejected from the penis. Symptoms of this condition may include the absence of sperm in ejaculation, or the presence of sperm in urine. Several medications can help reverse this problem.

Preventing Sexual Problems

Like so many of the complications discussed in this chapter, diabetes-related sexual problems can largely be avoided through good day-to-day health care that includes proper nutrition and adequate exercise. These measures—as well as regular examinations by your doctor—can help keep blood sugar levels low, maintain normal circulation, and otherwise enhance your health, preventing complications.

CONCLUSION

Most of the problems we have discussed in this chapter can be prevented, slowed, or alleviated by attention to proper diet, exercise, and a healthy lifestyle. If you have not been diligent about your healthcare and have experienced diabetes-related problems, you can help yourself by taking the preventative measures mentioned here. The majority of these problems are treatable. And once treated, their reoccurrence can sometimes be avoided by taking appropriate measures. But remember that prevention is always the best medicine.

CHAPTER EIGHT

Handling Special Situations

Self-care presents a particular challenge for people with diabetes. We have already discussed many circumstances that require you to learn new ways of coping. In a short time, these new approaches to your health care will become part of your everyday routine, and your diabetes control should improve. But there are two more situations that deserve special attention because they concern situations that take you out of your routine: sick days and traveling. Ordinary illnesses such as colds and flu require extraordinary care, and traveling requires extra attention to details. This chapter will cover the special care you require and the things you must remember to do when you are not feeling well and when you are traveling.

SICK DAYS

Physical and emotional stress can aggravate blood glucose levels. During stressful times, the body releases hormones that affect glucose levels in the body and can create problems with hyperglycemia. It is essential that you speak with your doctor and get specific instructions about managing your diabetes during sick days. By doing this *before* you get sick, you will be prepared to take good care of yourself.

Sick Day Recommendations

When you are developing a cold, flu, or other illness, your blood sugar levels will often be higher than usual because your body is trying to ward off infection. Since you can anticipate more problems with blood glucose control during these periods, it is a good idea to take the following precautions:

- Monitor your blood sugar *at least* four to five times a day when you are ill, especially before each meal, before bedtime, and during the night. Check your urine for ketones if your blood glucose is over 240 mg/dl. Record times and results of blood glucose and urine ketone monitoring so that you can give this information to your doctor as needed.

- Never stop taking your diabetes medication when you are sick unless your doctor advises you to do so—even if you are vomiting or not eating. You may need some adjustment in medication during illness. That's why frequent blood glucose monitoring and communication with your doctor during illness are so important.

- Many over-the-counter medications will affect blood glucose control. Check with your doctor or pharmacist before using any such medications. See Chapter 5 for more information about how different medications can affect diabetes control.

- Drink plenty of fluids in order to prevent dehydration. Try to drink at least eight ounces of fluid without sugar every hour during the day.

- If you are unable to follow your normal diet, supplement food intake by sipping beverages that contain sugar. Easy-to-digest foods that can supplement your usual diet include soups, gelatin with sugar, juice, eggs, and similar foods. If you are vomiting, sip a caffeine-free—not diet—soft drink or any drink containing sugar. Your dietitian can give you specific instructions for sick-day food and drinks in advance.

- Get plenty of rest and avoid exercise until you are well. Exercising when you are sick can increase blood glucose levels.

- Call your doctor for specific instructions if:
  - ❏ You do not improve in one day.
  - ❏ You have a temperature over 101°F.
  - ❏ You have vomiting or diarrhea that occurs more than once.
  - ❏ You have any problems with hypoglycemia during illness.
  - ❏ Your blood glucose is greater than 240 mg/dl or your ketone levels are moderate to high.
  - ❏ You have problems breathing.
  - ❏ You become progressively weaker.
  - ❏ You have any changes in your mental status.

TRAVELING AND DIABETES CONTROL

People with diabetes don't have to limit their travel, but traveling with diabetes does present special circumstances and challenges. Proper planning and preparation can help you meet those challenges. The following is a list of travel tips for people with diabetes:

- Research your destination to find out how to get medical care. If you are traveling to a country where people speak a language that you aren't familiar with, find out where you can find a doctor with whom you will be able to communicate. The International Association for Medical Assistance to Travelers can provide information on doctors who speak your primary language. The number is (716) 754-4883.

- Carry a letter signed—not stamped—by your doctor stating that you have diabetes and that you must carry insulin, medications, syringes, and other supplies with you. This will help you get through customs without problems. Take along prescriptions for your medications with the generic name of the medications identified. In addition, carry your doctor's telephone number with you.

- Carry your medication, supplies, testing materials, glucose tablets, and glucagon with you at all times. If you are traveling by plane, bus, or train, keep a carry-on with you. Do not check your insulin and supplies with your other bags! Protect your insulin, any other medications, testing strips, and supplies from extreme temperatures. Heat and cold can ruin them. Insulated travel kits are available at many pharmacies.

- Carry some snacks with you in case your meals are delayed.

- Always take more than enough diabetes medication and supplies with you in case your return home is delayed. Pack extra supplies in a separate carry-on suitcase.

- Call your local health department early and inquire about vaccinations that may be necessary or recommended for the area to which you are traveling.

- Check your blood sugar frequently while traveling. Four times a day is a good idea. Remember that there will be differences in your food intake, activity level, and sleep patterns.

- Wear your diabetes identification and carry a wallet card with you, too.

- Take cold remedies, diarrhea medication, and nausea medication with you.

- If you drive or sit for long periods of time while traveling, stretch your legs and walk around every one to two hours.

- If you are crossing time zones, ask your doctor or diabetes educator how to adjust your medication appropriately. Generally, crossing two or more time zones will require adjustments in your medication.

- If you must take injections during a flight, put only half as much air into the insulin bottle as you normally would. In-flight cabin pressure is lower, so you don't have to inject as much air into the insulin bottle when you draw up insulin.

- Try to keep meals and snack times as close to your regular schedule as possible.

- If you are taking insulin and you are more active than usual, be sure to decrease your insulin dose or increase your calories to compensate for the extra activity. Remember that some oral diabetes medications also have the potential to cause low blood sugar. Your doctor or diabetes educator can help you determine how your diet or medications should be adjusted.

- Be aware that different types and strengths of insulin are available in different countries. The type of insulin you normally take may not be available. Changing types and strengths of insulin can be very dangerous! That is one reason it is so important to take along more than enough diabetes medications and supplies. Some diabetes pills sold in the United States and Canada may not be available in other countries. Again, take extra medication with you.

- Be sure to get a traveler's health insurance policy in case you need medical care in a foreign country, as many domestic health-care policies do not cover illness in a foreign country.

CONCLUSION

As you can see, if you take the precautions and prepare as mentioned in this chapter, you can handle your sick days, and your activities will not be limited. In the back of this book, you will find a list of organizations that can help you with more information about sick days, travel, and other diabetes-related questions you may have.

Conclusion

If you have read this far, you have taken a major step toward gaining control of your diabetes. Now, take another deep breath, and put your newfound knowledge into practice. Look at your overall health and situation, and note the changes you must make in order to control your diabetes. If you start slowly by implementing one or two changes each week, you will bring about a great difference in your diabetes control. Evaluate your plan on an ongoing basis, and determine whether the changes you have made are working for you. If something is not working for you, choose an alternate plan.

Experience and research have shown that the tips, guidelines, and strategies presented in this book can be effective in helping you control diabetes and its complications. But remember that each person is different, and strategies that work for some may not be effective for everyone. This is why it is important for you to work with your physician and diabetes educator to fine-tune your plan.

As we have emphasized throughout this book, knowledge about diabetes and the technological advances in diabetes care are improving at a rate never before experienced. Keep yourself up-to-date about diabetes care and diabetes research. There is hope that one day a cure will be found for this disease. But until that day, it is essential that you stay in control and stay healthy.

Resources

Organizations

American Association of
   Diabetes Educators
100 West Monroe, 4th floor
Chicago, Illinois 60603
(800) 832-6874
http://www.aadenet.org

American Diabetes Association
1660 Duke Street
Alexandria, Virginia
22314-0592
(800) 232-3472 or (703) 549-1500
http://www.diabetes.org

American Dietetic Association
216 West Jackson Boulevard
Chicago, Illinois 60606-6995
(800) 366-1655
http://www.eatright.org

Canadian Diabetes Association
National Office
15 Toronto Street, suite 800
Toronto, ON M5C 2E3

(800) BANTING or
   (416) 363-3373
http://www.diabetes.ca/
   resources

The Canadian Dietetic
   Association
480 University Avenue, suite 601
Toronto, ON M5G 1V2
(416) 596-0857
http://www.dietitians.ca/
   resources

Canadian Medic Alert
   Foundation
250 Ferrand Drive, suite 301
Toronto, ON M3C 2T9
(800) 668-6381

The Centers for Disease Control
   and Prevention
National Center for Chronic
   Disease Prevention and
   Health Promotion, Division
   of Diabetes Translation

4770 Buford Highway, NE
Mail Stop 10-K
Atlanta, Georgia 30341-3724
(770) 488-5000
http://www.cdc.gov/nccdphp/
ddt/ddthome.htm

The International Association
for Medical Assistance to
Travelers
(716) 754-4883

International Diabetic Athletes
Association
1931 East Rovey Avenue
Phoenix, Arizona 85016
(602) 433-2113

Juvenile Diabetes Foundation
120 Wall Street
19th Floor
New York, New York 10005
(800) JDF-CURE

National Diabetes Information
Clearinghouse
1 Information Way
Bethesda, Maryland 20892-3560
(301) 654-3327

Publications and Videotapes

Armchair Fitness Videos
(Chair Exercise Videos)
(800) 453-6280

Diabetes Interview Magazine
3715 Balboa Street
San Francisco, California
94121-9836
www.diabetesworld.com
Fax: (800) 324-9434
(800) 234-1218

*Diabetes Self-Management
Magazine*
Published by: R.A. Rapaport
Publishing Company
P.O. Box 52890
Boulder, Colorado 80322
(800) 234-0923

The Diabetic Reader Newsletter
Prana Publications and
Paraphernalia
5623 Matilija Avenue
Van Nuys, California 91401
(800) 735-7726

Sit and Be Fit Video Series
(Chair Exercise Exercises)
Collage Video
(800) 433-6769

References

American Association of Diabetes Educators. *New Approaches to Type II Diabetes: Practical Clinical Applications of the Latest Developments in the Management of Type II Diabetes.* Booklet from AADE seminar held in Panama City, Florida, June 1997.

American Diabetes Association. "Clinical Practice Recommendations 1997." *Diabetes Care Supplement 1* (1997), 20.

American Diabetes Association. "Information about Metformin, an Oral Medication for People with Type 2 diabetes." *American Diabetes Association Newsletter* (May 4, 1995).

American Diabetes Association. Position Statement. "Nutrition Recommendations and Principles for People with Diabetes Mellitus." *Diabetes Care* (1994) 17(5):519–522.

American Diabetes Association. "Report of the Expert Committee on the Diagnosis and Classification of Diabetes Mellitus." *Diabetes Care* (1997) 20(7), 1183–1197.

American Diabetes Association. "Yet another Pill for Type 2s." *The Diabetes Advisor* (1998) 6(3):1.

Bristol-Myers Squibb Company. Package insert for Glucophage (metformin hydrochloride tablets), 1998.

Dawson K. "Oral Hypoglycaemic Agent Therapy in Diabetes 1997." Canadian Diabetes Association Web site http://www.diabetes.ca. Last update, September 22, 1998.

Diabetes Medical Practice Guidelines. State of Florida Agency for Health Care Administration in consultation with the Diabetes Guideline Advisory Committee. January 16, 1998.

Foster-Powell, K. and Miller, J.B. International Tables of Glycemic Index. *American Journal of Clinical Nutrition* (1995) 62:871S–93S.

Eriksson J. et al. "Resistance Training in the Treatment of Non-Insulin-Dependent Diabetes Mellitus." *Int. J. Sports Medicine* (1997) 18:242–246.

"The Expert Committee on the Diagnosis and Classification of Diabetes Mellitus." *Diabetes Care* (1997) 20(7):1183–1196.

Foster-Powell, K. and J.B. Miller. "International Tables of Glycemic Index." *American Journal of Clinical Nutrition* (1995) 62:871S–893S.

Hamilton, C.C., P. Geil, and J.W. Anderson. "Management of Obesity in Diabetes Mellitus." *Diabetes Educator* (1992) 18(5):407–410.

Holler, H.J. and J.G. Pastors. *Diabetes Medical Nutrition Therapy.* American Dietetic Association/American Diabetes Association, 1997.

Ivy, J. "Role of Exercise Training in the Prevention and Treatment of Insulin Resistance and Non-Insulin-Dependent Diabetes Mellitus." *Sports Medicine* (1997) 24(5):321–336.

Jenkins, D.J.A. et al. "Glycemic Index of Foods: A Physiological Basis for Carbohydrate Exchange." *American Journal of Clinical Nutrition* (1981) 34:362–366.

Oki, J. and W. Isley. "Rethinking New and Old Diabetes Drugs for Type 2 Diabetes." *Practical Diabetology* (1997) 16 (3):27–40.

Parke-Davis Pharmaceutical. *Locked Out of Control.* Rezulin pamphlet, 1997.

Peragallo-Dittko, V., K. Godley, and J. Meyer. *A Core Curriculum for Diabetes Education*, 2nd ed. Chicago: American Association of Diabetes Educators and the AADE Education Research Foundation, 1993.

Pharmacia and Upjohn. *Erectile Dysfunction: Asking the Right Questions.* Pharmacia and Upjohn, 1997.

Pi-Sunyer, F.X. "Weight and Non-Insulin-Dependent Diabetes Mellitus." *American Journal of Clinical Nutrition* (1996) 63(suppl): 4265–4295.

Salmeron, J. et al. "Dietary Fiber, Glycemic Load, and Risk of Non-Insulin Dependent Diabetes Mellitus in Women." *Journal of the American Medical Association* (1997) 474–477.

Satcher, D. *Diabetes: A Serious Public Health Problem at A Glance.* US Department of Health and Human Services, Public Health Service, Centers for Disease Control and Prevention, 1996.

Wallberg-Henriksson H., J. Rincon, and J.R. Zierath. "Exercise in the Management of Non-Insulin-Dependent diabetes mellitus." *Sports Medicine* (1998) 25(1):25–35.

Weil, R. *Exercising with Complications: Diabetes Self-Management* (September/October 1997) 14(5):61–68.

Wolever, T.M.S et al. "Beneficial Effect of a Low Glycemic Index Diet in Type 2 Diabetes." *Diabetic Medicine* (1992) 9:451–458.

Zonszein J. "The Diabetic Stomach." *Practical Diabetology* (1997) 16(2):4–8.

Conversion Tables

As explained in Chapter 1, in the United States, blood glucose, cholesterol, and triglyercide levels are expressed in milligrams per deciliter (mg/dl). However, the rest of the world expresses these levels in millimoles per liter (mmol/L). The following tables will allow you to instantly convert your test results from one system to another. (For easy conversion formulas, see the inset on page 13.)

Glucose Levels

(mg/dl) = (mmol/L)		(mg/dl) = (mmol/L)		(mg/dl) = (mmol/L)		(mg/dl) = (mmol/L)	
70	3.89	115	6.39	160	8.89	205	11.39
75	4.17	120	6.67	165	9.17	210	11.67
80	4.44	125	6.94	170	9.44	215	11.94
85	4.72	130	7.22	175	9.72	220	12.22
90	5.00	135	7.50	180	10.00	225	12.50
95	5.28	140	7.78	185	10.28	230	12.78
100	5.56	145	8.06	190	10.56	235	13.06
105	5.83	150	8.33	195	10.83	240	13.33
110	6.11	155	8.61	200	11.11	245	13.61

Cholesterol Levels

(mg/dl) = (mmol/L)		(mg/dl) = (mmol/L)		(mg/dl) = (mmol/L)		(mg/dl) = (mmol/L)	
35	0.90	90	2.32	145	3.75	200	5.17
40	1.03	95	2.45	150	3.88	205	5.30
45	1.16	100	2.58	155	4.01	210	5.43
50	1.29	105	2.71	160	4.13	215	5.56
55	1.42	110	2.84	165	4.26	220	5.68
60	1.55	115	2.97	170	4.39	225	5.81
65	1.68	120	3.10	175	4.52	230	5.94
70	1.81	125	3.23	180	4.65	235	6.07
75	1.94	130	3.36	185	4.78	240	6.20
80	2.07	135	3.49	190	4.91	245	6.33
85	2.20	140	3.62	195	5.04	250	6.45

Triglyceride Levels

(mg/dl) = (mmol/L)		(mg/dl) = (mmol/L)		(mg/dl) = (mmol/L)		(mg/dl) = (mmol/L)	
150	1.69	190	2.15	230	2.60	270	3.05
155	1.75	195	2.20	235	2.66	275	3.11
160	1.81	200	2.26	240	2.71	280	3.16
165	1.86	205	2.32	245	2.77	285	3.22
170	1.92	210	2.37	250	2.82	290	3.28
175	1.98	215	2.43	255	2.88	295	3.33
180	2.03	220	2.49	260	2.94	300	3.39
185	2.09	225	2.54	265	2.99	305	3.44

Index